Understanding Women's Recovery From Illness and Trauma

Margaret H. Kearney

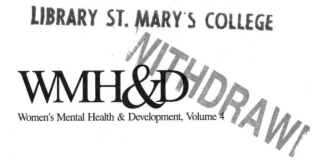

WMH&D

Women's Mental Health & Development, Volume 4

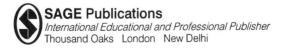
SAGE Publications
International Educational and Professional Publisher
Thousand Oaks   London   New Delhi

For information:

SAGE Publications, Inc.
2455 Teller Road
Thousand Oaks, California 91320
E-mail: order@sagepub.com

SAGE Publications Ltd.
6 Bonhill Street
London EC2A 4PU
United Kingdom

SAGE Publications India Pvt. Ltd.
M-32 Market
Greater Kailash I
New Delhi 110 048 India

Printed in the United States of America

Library of Congress Cataloging-in-Publication Data

Kearney, Margaret H.
Understanding women's recovery from illness and trauma / by
    Margaret H. Kearney
        p. cm.— (Women's mental health and development; v. 4)
    Includes index.
    ISBN 0-7619-0558-8 (cloth)
    ISBN 0-7619-0559-6 (paperback)
    1. Women—Health and hygiene. 2. Women—Diseases—Social aspects.
3. Women—Diseases—Psychological aspects. 4. Social medicine.
5. Psychic trauma. 6. Catastrophic illness—Psychological aspects.
I. Title. II. Series.
RA564.85 .K425   1999
616'.0082—dc21   99-6104

This book is printed on acid-free paper.

99 00 01 02 03 04 05   7 6 5 4 3 2 1

Acquiring Editor: Jim Nageotte
Editorial Assistant: Heidi Van Middlesworth
Production Editor: Wendy Westgate
Production Assistant: Nevair Kabakian
Cover Designer: Ravi Balasuriya

Contents

Series Editor's Introduction

One of the outcomes of the women's movement is the increasing attention to women's experiences of and responses to health issues across the life span. Just as women's development differs from that of men, the types of illnesses, treatments, and the overall impact on women's sense of self, relationships, family, and work also differ. Although research in the areas of women's health is burgeoning, there are still many health care providers who are not attuned to gender differences in the nature and types of illness experiences. Clinicians can learn about how women restructure their identity, relationships, and life patterns in response to health-related events from a comprehensive overview of the research to-date and from women's personal stories.

In Volume 4 of the Sage Women's Mental Health and Development series, Margaret H. Kearney synthesizes existing theories about women's experiences of health crises, recovery, and growth from different disciplines with personal stories of women into a cohesive phase model that allows us to provide meaningful support, understanding, and care for women undergoing health transformations. Working with Dr. Kearney on this volume has positively affected my clinical work: Teaching her transformation model to clients and their families has provided a guiding framework for understanding the difficult and challenging process of transformation. This process involves letting go of pre-illness or trauma assumptions about who we are, what we can do, and how things are "supposed" to be so that we can develop a more flexible self paradigm that allows us to shift roles, responsibilities, and identities. Husbands, friends, parents, and children face the same challenges to their views of "the way things are supposed to be."

Dr. Kearney presents her material in a way that allows us to view differences in the perspectives of the meaning of health, illness, and treatment through the lenses of culture, ethnicity, socioeconomic class, and spirituality, as well as consideration of the impact of one's unique personal history and environmental stressors. This aspect of women's development is critical to our understanding and treatment of women in all stages of life, given the reported prevalence of depression, eating disorders, cancer, heart disease, chronic illness, and strokes. The author brings her 25 years of women's health nurse practitioner experience in urban, rural, poor, and wealthy areas of the United States to this commendable task. Researchers, clinicians of all disciplines, and academicians interested in women's issues can all benefit from this thoughtful, clarifying volume.

The Editorial Board and I believe this book is an invaluable companion to the other volumes in the series. Forthcoming volumes will deal with women and cancer and women's psychopharmacology.

Barbara F. Okun, Ph.D.
Northeastern University

For Emily and Paul

Preface

Through struggle and surrender, ill people paradoxically grow more resolute in self as they adapt to impairment. . . They believe in their inner strength as their bodies crumble. They transcend their bodies as they surrender control. . . With this stance comes a sense of resolution and an awareness of timing. They know when to struggle and when to flow into surrender. They grow impervious to social meanings, including being devalued. They can face the unknown without fear while remaining themselves. At this point, chronically ill people may find themselves in the ironic position of giving solace and comfort to the healthy.

--Charmaz, 1995, p. 675

LISTENING TO WOMEN ABOUT ILLNESS

Women in pain, whether physical, emotional, or spiritual, make up much of the clientele in counseling caseloads. Counselors spend many hours eliciting and listening to women's stories of how their lives and views of themselves have changed as they have suffered losses, setbacks, and surprises along life's path. Some life transitions or untoward events--such as divorce, bereavement, infertility, or parenting difficulties--are common enough that counselors have plentiful literature to draw from in helping these women and are able to recognize common responses and stages of recovery and healing.

The goal of this book is to provide similar support for counseling of women suffering illness or recovering from trauma. It offers real-life experiential information from women themselves. I also theorize about common threads of experience of women who have moved through these difficulties and reached a point of resolution. The theory presented in Chapter 2, which is rooted not in hypothetical "armchair" speculation but in a careful analysis of over 100 studies of many hundreds of women, is reiterated in the subsequent chapters focusing on particular situations of illness and trauma. Counselors may find this model useful for their work with women in health-related transitions. The women quoted in the book provide insights into how they found strength and resilience in integrating great loss and devastation into their lives.

This book is written by a nurse and draws predominantly from nursing research literature. It explores and synthesizes theoretical viewpoints on health arising from nurses' interest in patients' experiences and their research methods drawn from anthropology and medical sociology. It may be useful to researchers who are interested in a collection of small studies of health experiences. Yet the main purpose here is to offer insights for clinicians. I bring to this project many years of experience as a women's health nurse practitioner; my clinical work has served as a testing ground for the ideas in this book. Nurse researchers have made important contributions to understanding the experiences of health and illness, which should be disseminated beyond our profession. Although nurses focus on prevention and treatment of physical and mental illness, like counselors, our broad focus is on supporting individuals toward their optimal level of wellness and growth within their unique life contexts. Therefore, the goal of this book is to offer a synthesis of ideas from nurses' and others' observations of women's illness experiences that will be useful to counselors and others working directly with women undergoing health changes.

Although nurse researchers and other scientists are conscientiously seeking to remedy this deficit, women marginalized by poverty, language and cultural difference, and illness itself have been inadequately studied and heard in past years and as a result are less visible in this book than I would like. Context is indeed critical to every woman's view of herself and her possibilities. What illness means, what recovery consists of, what a woman with a disability should be doing within a culture or society, how much a woman should attend to her own rather than her family's needs, the role of the environment and the spiritual world in disease all are defined differently within diverse age groups, families, social worlds, and cultural traditions. In my nursing practice with women of all income ranges and educational levels and in my nursing research with women who are substance users and survivors of domestic violence, I have gained sensitivity to the importance of ethnic, cultural, and socioeconomic differences in women's understandings of their lives and relationships.

Unfortunately, due to lack of available research, this book will not answer all the important questions about how diversity affects illness experience. Any effort like this one to generalize about experience must smooth over the bumps and irregularities of unique life stories and pass over the minute differences in personal histories and conditions of women's lives. One can only tell a few parts of a story at a time, which flattens out a three-dimensional life into a line or diagram. Although this book brings together many studies of many kinds of illness and trauma experiences, we can only speculate about other unstudied situations. Many questions will remain.

One question this book will not answer is whether women's illness experience resembles men's experience. Certainly, women's roles and relationships and how women are socialized from infancy to understand themselves and their place in the world create different experiences of illness and loss, but the focus here is on women's stories in themselves rather than on contrasts or comparisons. Another unanswered question is how women in the United States and Canada resemble women from other regions. With a very few exceptions, this book is based on studies of North American English-speaking women.

THE POWER OF STORIES TOLD TOGETHER

As will become obvious in the next chapter, there is a surprising dearth of large-scale research on women's health problems. With the exception of health problems affecting reproduction, neither the physical manifestations and consequences nor the psychological impact of women's illness has been studied in depth until very recently. The studies that exist are often limited to women of racial and ethnic majority status. Major new initiatives also are limited to a focus on menopause and related health problems. Therefore, we are unable to make broad-based statements about "what happens to women with multiple sclerosis" or "the psychological effects of arthritis for women."

Nor would this meet the needs of counselors who see individual women, one at a time, and seek to understand their unique experiences. We respond to women as they seek to put illness into context and readjust their lives and goals around their changing health. This book aims to give therapists and other professionals a head start--an opportunity to hear from many women who have told their stories to researchers, who in turn have organized the stories into a cohesive set of findings.

This book is a synthesis of qualitative research: systematic study of human experience using text, visual observation, the spoken word, and other "live" sources as data, rather than converting personal experiences into numbers and using statistical analysis to come to conclusions. Qualitative researchers study "lived reality," the subjective experience of being in a particular situation at a particular time (Munhall, 1995). This approach recognizes that the values and beliefs of both researcher and researched will affect the goals and outcomes of study and that the findings of such research are cocreated by scientist and participant. The product of a qualitative research study is a description of an experience, in theoretical terms or in the form of narrative or themes.

The epistemological tenet here is that personal stories have truth value that is different than that of large-sample survey research with high statistical power. I make no claim of generalizability of the experiences portrayed here, nor do the small studies from which these women's voices are drawn rely on random sampling or large numbers. The rigor of this text-based (as opposed to numbers-based) science is found not in random sampling or statistical compensation for chance findings but in the researcher's adherence to a specific interpretive approach, a meticulous faithfulness to the participants' perspective during a systematic analysis of meanings. The value of small-scale, in-depth research is not in its applicability to large groups but in the relevance of the experiences portrayed herein to the reader's own professional needs. A woman's statement or a theoretical conclusion drawn from many statements is meaningful and valid if it has what Glaser and Strauss (1967) called "fit" with the reader's experience and "grab" in its recognizability, logical coherence, and believability.

Qualitative research can attempt to answer the "why" and "how" questions of human responses to illness. Listening to 6 women can yield more about their lived experience of suffering and processes of self-transformation than can reading an excellent statistical report on the effectiveness of a medical treatment or the frequency of depression or anxiety. Readers rather than computerized analyses judge the significance of this type of research, which is designed to gather vivid and meaningful examples of human experience on a particular topic.

WHAT IS GROUNDED-THEORY RESEARCH?

This book is built on studies that employed grounded theory, a form of qualitative research aimed at discovering theory about human perceptions and actions (Glaser & Strauss, 1967). The goal is not to simply describe the essence of an experience for a group of people but to make theoretical conclusions about how people respond to this situation and how the experience changes over time. This makes it well-suited to the process of illness and recovery. Theory discovered in this way is systematically developed from experiential information using a technique of constant comparison, drawing theoretical ideas from the original data and expanding and modifying these ideas by constant comparison of all data sources to each other.

Grounded theorists develop samples for research not by restricting themselves to a homogeneous group but by seeking to maximize the variation within a sample. Theoretical sampling involves seeking out new situations to observe and new participants to speak with who can help clarify the areas of the emerging theory that are still unclear. The researcher continues to collect data until no new information is being discovered. The usual result is a theoretical model of a social-psychological process shared by a variety of participants in a particular life situation and the conditions and contingencies that affect individuals' progress through the phases of the process (Strauss & Corbin, 1990). Using a theory of recovery from a particular illness or loss, clinicians can begin to predict the phases of recovery and the potential obstacles or resources, and help clients move toward positive outcomes.

Here, we will take the act of bringing together women's stories one step further by providing an overarching theoretical framework that can be used to place women's statements along a continuum of change. For this book, a higher-level grounded theory known as *grounded formal theory* (Strauss, 1987) was developed. It is presented in Chapter 2. This is the result of analysis of the many single grounded-theory studies presented in the later chapters to find a process that all the groups studied have in common. It was developed using the same steps of constant comparison and theoretical sampling that the original studies used, but the "participants" were not individual women but the hundred-plus individual articles, books, or dissertations. The resulting theory is of necessity very general, but its basic concepts are important to any woman struggling to come to terms with illness or trauma. With this simple model in mind, counselors can be alert to important issues and support women as they work through their unique and particular losses.

In bookstores and magazines can be found many stories of women's personal journeys through illness or misfortune. These books are mainly by or about women who were writers or public figures before they became ill. They have value in their own right, but they are not drawn on here because they are not produced by systematic research on ordinary people. Nonetheless, these single-person accounts echo all the components of the processes described here and can serve as in-depth examples. Among professional publications, there are also other book-length collections of studies of women's illness experiences (e.g., Munhall, 1994, 1995; Young-Mason, 1997).

This book does not aim to teach counselors new techniques or even new ways of applying old skills. Rather, it is designed to provide windows into aspects of women's experience that counselors may not encounter on a regular basis. Whenever feasible, direct quotations from women as cited by grounded theory researchers are used to demonstrate important components of illness experience. The result is a story that makes sense and that can be used to understand and support women who are living through it. This is a tale of reckoning with hard truths over time and finding ways to reconcile these losses with the ongoing priorities of women's lives. Reckoning and reconciling form a framework of illness recovery that produces not only accommodation to the daily demands of poor health but growth toward a new idea of self-actualization.

Acknowledgments

This book was made possible by more than 100 qualitative researchers in nursing, counseling, and the health sciences. Their publications and dissertations are the platform on which this work is built, and any misinterpretations are mine alone. Thanks also to Boston College for a Faculty Research Expense Grant that funded a summer of library work, and to my editors, Barbara Okun and Jim Nageotte, without whose support and excellent judgment this book would not be what it is. I am continually grateful to the women and men who told their stories of illness, pain, and healing to the researchers cited in this book, and to all those who continue patiently to instruct their health care providers about the experience of illness.

1

Why Listen to Women

The Social and Political Context
of Women's Health and Illness

WHAT WE DON'T KNOW

Women may live longer than men, but men appear to be healthier. Their mortality advantage has been declining since the 1970s, but women still live an average of 7 years longer than men. However, during their longer lives, women receive more treatment than do men for acute illnesses, mental health problems, and nonfatal chronic illnesses, have one third more physician visits, use more prescription and nonprescription drugs, and lose more time from work due to minor disabilities (Stanton, 1995). They are more likely to be affected by diseases of the very old such as Alzheimer's disease and osteoporosis (Weisman & Cassard, 1994). Women occupy 75% of nursing home beds and receive the majority of Medicare and Medicaid funds (Friedman, 1994).

Yet until recently, women have been excluded from much biomedical research other than that focusing on reproduction. Their capacities for understanding health-related information, accuracy of self-knowledge about their own symptoms and problems, and abilities to control their emotions and rise above dependent roles have been doubted by their professional care providers. Only in the past two decades have women begun to achieve voice and control over their roles in health care systems. In entering the arena as physicians, health care advocates, and policy makers, women have brought new appreciation for individual experience as a valid source of knowledge, for representation of diversity of all kinds as important to decision making, and for professional and personal relationships as part of healing. In this changing context, the voices of women have a new power and authority. This book is an effort to contribute to better understanding of women's illness experiences.

The Shortcomings of Empirical Research

Women have indeed been systematically excluded from large-scale studies of medical problems and treatment, for reasons both scientific and social. At the turn of the century, most women's illnesses were thought to be due to their hormonal changes and reproductive problems. Most of their complaints were considered the product of emotional instability or their lot as childbearers and not serious enough for intervention unless reproductive capacity was affected. Many women accepted the prevailing advice to avoid vigorous activity and take particular care of themselves during the vulnerable time of menstruation to avoid injuring their reproductive organs. Victorian modesty prevented discussion of intimate health problems or examination of women's bodies even with trusted physicians. For the few women who saw a need and took the risk to speak up for themselves and their gender, lesser education and exclusion from most professions contributed to their inability to be heard in circles of power (LaRosa & Pinn, 1993). Feminist historians have suggested that women were placated rather than treated more definitively by physicians because as businessmen, they recognized that women were their best customers and would keep coming back (Ehrenreich & English, 1977). As recently as 1993, women still received more first-time prescriptions for psychotropic drugs than did men, although male physicians were more likely than female physicians to give psychotropic drugs to women (Taggart, McCammon, Allred, Horner, & May, 1993).

The diseases women were expected to have--sexual problems, breast cancer, mental health problems, and menopause--were for many years deemed too indelicate or too insignificant for consideration by medical researchers. The exception was pregnancy-related problems, which were considered important to society and the impetus for many cruel and permanently harmful treatments in hope of improving childbearing capacity or pregnancy outcomes (Ehrenreich & English, 1977). The diseases that were the focus of research, mainly the leading causes of death, such as heart disease, were not thought to be important in women because women were not severely affected until later in life than men. Women's illnesses were followed in observational studies, such as the Framingham Heart Study (e.g., Allen & Blumenthal, 1998) and the Nurses' Health Study (e.g., Fuchs, 1999), but experimental research was lacking (LaRosa & Pinn, 1993). Yet the major causes of death to women are not gender specific, with the exception of breast cancer. Heart disease and AIDS are two leading killers of women, and in both cases, women were excluded from the initial treatment research, which may have contributed to women's lower survival rates from these illnesses (Weisman & Cassard, 1994).

Many illnesses have been thought to be affected by women's reproductive systems and hormones, and therefore women's responses were considered too unpredictable for controlled studies. Some problems, such as heart disease, were infrequent enough in young and middle-aged women that including women in studies would require much larger samples and greater expense. In the case of AIDS, women affected by the disease were predominantly poor women of color involved with drug use and as a consequence, had little voice in the activist movement dominated by gay men. Yet AIDS is the leading cause of death in women of reproductive age in some parts of the United States (Weisman & Cassard, 1994).

Studies involving medications or invasive treatments very often excluded women of childbearing age for fear of causing harm to fetuses (LaRosa & Pinn, 1993). This protectionism, although it originated in good-faith efforts to protect vulnerable research participants from being harmed by research, does not account for the pervasive unwillingness of researchers to trust a woman's assertions that she would not or could not become pregnant during a research experiment. Nor does it account for the lack of major research initiatives before the 1980s on problems unique to women (Mastroianni, Faden, & Federman, 1994).

The consequence is that research conclusions derived from studies of men are applied to women without scientific basis (Angell, 1993), and occasionally treatment is denied women because there is no evidence that it will be effective. One female scientist recalled that when a male colleague commented that thanks to recent research on caffeine and heart disease, "I guess our hearts are safe if we have a cup of coffee," she replied, "*Your* heart may be safe; I have no idea about the safety of my heart! That study was conducted on over 45,000 men" (Stanton, 1995, p. 3). In many more serious situations, medications and treatments tested only on men have been given to women only to find after the fact that women had very different outcomes. For example, angioplasty, a very common surgical treatment for heart disease, has poorer outcomes for women than for men, for reasons not yet well understood (Weisman & Cassard, 1994).

Undervalued, Disbelieved

The past absence of women in science and medicine has contributed to the lack of attention to women's health issues and, until recently, the lack of dialog about how women could be included in mixed-gender studies without undue risk or scientific compromise. Until approximately 1970, women in general did not have the social and cultural authority to be heard (LaRosa & Pinn, 1993). The underrepresentation of women in the sciences has mirrored the discrediting of women's intellects and opinions and the silencing of women's voices in many venues of society. The alternative forms of experiencing and knowing articulated by women (Belenky, 1997; Gilligan, 1993) have only recently been granted credibility as scientific approaches and as sources of valid symptom-related information.

Although most patients are women and more surgical procedures are done on women than on men (cesarean section and hysterectomy, for example, are two of the six most common surgeries), informed consent for medical procedures has been heavily influenced by paternalism and male authority. Until recently, husbands were often included in consent for procedures on their wives, presumably because men were thought to better understand medical technicalities (Annas, 1994). Furthermore, women's understandings of their own bodies have been belittled in their communication with doctors. Until recently, women have been denied information on the full range of available options for treatment for diseases such as breast cancer and perimenopausal bleeding, making them vulnerable to unnecessary mastectomies and hysterectomies. These may be expedient cures of illness but have lasting implications for women's quality of life.

Doctors have not listened well to women. The communication between physicians and their patients reveals striking differences when gender is considered. The doctor-patient relationship in general has long been intentionally asymmetrical, with control over the interaction in the hands of the physician. This control has been thought necessary to enable the doctor to gather information and perform examinations efficiently to provide the best diagnostic and therapeutic service to patients. Yet a more mutual level of participation is important when critical information is held by patients, when patients are expected to play key roles in performing treatments essential to recovery, and when physicians dispense information and need to verify the patient's understanding (West, 1984).

Nonetheless, physicians interrupt patients far more than the reverse, except when both patient and doctor are white males, or when the physician is a woman. Female patients and male and female patients of color are interrupted more and ask fewer questions than white male patients, except when the physician is a woman. Medical information is most likely to be misheard or misunderstood in the absence of two-way communication, and therefore, women and patients of color are disadvantaged in many medical encounters (West, 1984). Doctors do not hesitate to tell women what to do, however. Female patients and patients of higher social class receive more information from physicians, which has been linked to women's ability to elicit warm responses from providers and providers' assumptions that higher-class patients are better educated and more invested in health (Hall, Roter, & Katz, 1988). Yet the unfortunate reality is that in the United States, women are much less likely than men to be financially well-off, and professionals may therefore assume that most women have less education and less ability to understand (or motivation to use) health-related information.

When the physician is a woman, the picture changes somewhat. Female physicians establish a more equal exchange with patients (West, 1984), spend more time and talk more with both male and female patients, order preventive screening tests more often, and are rated more highly in patient satisfaction (Johnston, 1996). Women who choose nurse-midwives over obstetricians for their childbirth health care often cite the (usually female) nurse-midwives' willingness to listen to women's concerns and wishes, and their respect for privacy and gentleness when performing pelvic and other examinations (Welch, 1996). Yet in many specialties, female physicians remain in the minority, decreasing the likelihood that women patients will have access to health care providers who will grant them an equitable role in their own health care.

Women Outside the Privileged Center

The most serious dearth of health information pertains to women of color, immigrants, the very elderly, lesbians, and the poor. Research on the needs and best treatment of women who are not white, well-educated, socioeconomically advantaged, or have access to high-quality health care is virtually nonexistent (Rosser, 1994).

Categories such as race can be artificial distinctions. Race is now accepted to be as much a social, historical, and political entity as a biological distinction. For example, the number of races in the world has been described as from three to dozens, whether using skin color, biological markers, or genealogy. For 40 years, UNESCO has promoted the policy that "race is less a biological fact than a social myth" (Gamble & Blustein, 1994, p. 177). Yet, black women in the United States continue to suffer more from conditions such as hypertension and infant mortality than their white counterparts, and black women are much less likely than are white women to receive surgical treatments even when their disease state is similar (Lavizzo-Mourey & Grisso, 1994). Most health policy analysts now agree that social class and race must be considered together when studying health differences, as socioeconomic hardship and oppression are often more powerful than race in explaining illness (Gamble & Blustein, 1994). Like race, ethnicity is subject to faulty construction, as when all Asians or Native Americans are assumed to be similar, whether their origins are China or Hawaii, or Florida or Alaska.

Although inclusion of diverse groups in health research is essential, the assumption of difference and the design of medical research based on difference can cause more harm than good for women of color. Historically, explanations for black women's health problems have been based on low intelligence, an inborn tendency to promiscuity, or lack of motivation, when white women's problems were explained based on socially acceptable behaviors. Today, osteoporosis is still considered a greater risk for white and Asian than for African American women, and black women have been sidelined in educational campaigns to prevent osteoporosis. Yet age and gender, not race, are the main predictors of this disease. Weight, smoking, and other factors have not been sufficiently examined when African American women were assumed to have biological protection (Gamble & Blustein, 1994). Researchers are now being advised to describe study participants by self-identified ethnicity as well as many other important distinctions including socioeconomic status, but not to generalize about why differences occur without careful analysis of the many potential influences on health (Mastroianni et al., 1994).

Diverse Meanings of Illness

More research is needed on how cultural differences affect health and health care. Cultures, religions, and ethnic traditions vary in their understandings of how the body works, how the body and mind relate, the meanings of health and illness, the role of family in decision-making, and the appropriate approaches to healing. These differences are compounded by a profound distrust of the biomedical "establishment" by many women, including Native Americans, lesbians, people of color, and immigrants, who based on valid historical examples of medical abuse and decades of prejudice in health care interactions are understandably reluctant to participate in medical studies or heed their results. For example, women of color have been forcibly sterilized as recently as the 1970s (Gamble & Blustein, 1994). Doctor-patient interactions and requests to participate in research, often already laden with medical paternalism, are especially threatening to cultural minority women.

Kleinman (1988), a physician who has spent years studying patients' experiences of illness in various cultures, has long held that health care must address not only the symptoms and progression of the disease but the impact of the illness and its meanings within the life of the patient. Symptoms are experienced and described differently in different cultural and social groups. For example, in industrialized Western culture, a symptom such as stomach pain is an indication of disrupted mechanics of body function, and its causes are based on anatomy, physiology, and biomedical disease. Our bodies are considered to be independent of their surroundings, the sum of interacting parts. By contrast, in traditional Asian and Native American cultures the body may be experienced as a microcosm of the larger natural world and symptoms as a reflection of larger imbalances. Stomach pain might be a sign of moral weakness, blocked life energy, or disharmony in social interaction. In the United States, local meanings may be more useful than wider cultural ones, as subcultures exist within urban and rural communities, immigrant groups, or African American and Latino American folk traditions. The task of helpers is to elicit the meaning of symptoms as they occur within a specific life context.

Moral and spiritual meanings of illness may cause much of the distress suffered by the ill. Illness viewed as a sign of sin, punishment, or alienation from God may bring great suffering. In Western societies, victims of disease are often blamed (and blame themselves) for their own conditions, implying moral weakness as a cause and moral fortitude as a cure. For example, persons with heart problems who do not stop smoking or eating high-fat foods are judged less morally worthy than others who make sweeping reforms in response to their diagnoses.

Personal and social meanings of illness include how the problem disrupts a woman's past history, anticipated life course, family and community, and her identity and sense of self. For an adolescent wanting to be popular and eat pizza and ice cream with her friends, diabetes is a different experience than for a single mother who is considering teaching her preschool children how to revive her from insulin shock. Women's judgments about the significance of their illnesses and their subsequent responses are rooted in their own lives and biographies. Helpers must attempt to grasp and work within their patients' value systems if they are to offer useful relief of suffering (Kleinman, 1988).

Recent legislation has mandated the inclusion of women and racial and ethnic minorities in biomedical research so that the findings will include valid evidence of whether the factors under study affect women or racial or ethnic minority groups differently than white male participants. Yet much work is still needed before the methods of scientific research, the questions that are asked, and the values underlying the studies arise from and respect the diversity of the people being studied. The specific context and meaning of scientific research within the many communities of participants must be considered before researchers can engage the participation of individuals who have long been silent and invisible within the biomedical realm (Mastroianni et al., 1994).

In sum, due to historical, political, social, and cultural inequities, women's illnesses have been devalued and their opinions and experiences disregarded, their participation in the medical community and as patients has been restricted, and their needs and treatments have been inadequately studied. Yet women are the largest consumers of health care and of federal dollars spent on health.

WHY LISTEN NOW

Women's Self-Help and Advocacy Reaches Maturity

The timing of this effort coincides with recent shifts in public recognition of women's health care needs. Although advocates for women's health have had important local influences through history, in the 1960s, a widespread movement of self-help and advocacy arose that brought about permanent changes in understanding of women's health needs. The Boston Women's Health Collective (1985), producers of the pivotal work, *Our Bodies, Ourselves*, were among the visible and vocal change agents working for empowerment of women in the arena of health. Although the feminist health centers that arose in the early 1970s are less visible today or have been replaced by women's health specialty practices, the most important and lasting effect of that era of women's rights was a new policy-level and practitioner-level acceptance of women's right to be informed and active in health care interactions (Eagan, 1994).

An eventual product of this consciousness-raising and of the dramatic increase in female physicians and scientists that accompanied the wider women's movement was the greater attention to women's health issues in federal research funding priorities, culminating recently in the formation of the Office of Research on Women's Health within the National Institutes for Health (Mastroianni et al., 1994), and the Women's Health Initiative, a huge study of the impact of postmenopausal treatments on women's heart disease and other problems. Despite this long-overdue allocation of attention and resources to women's health, there is disagreement among physicians about the merit of focusing on women's health issues as unique from men's, especially when women are in fact the majority in the United States, and few of their life-threatening illnesses are unique to women. A prominent female medical journal editor has argued that research studies large enough to include women of all ethnic variations are prohibitively costly and that making women's health a specialty ensures that women will remain on the margins of research, as exceptions rather than the rule (Angell, 1993).

At the grass-roots level, important changes already have occurred in ordinary health-care encounters. Women's call for a less interventionist approach to childbirth has moved childbirth education from back rooms and basements to hospital conference rooms, and birth centers and anesthesia options are commonplace in most parts of the country for women with access to high-quality care. Women have made breast cancer a central public concern, have begun to claim menopause as a normal developmental process rather than the end of womanhood, and have made female-controlled contraception the norm. The movement for patients' rights arose in large part from women's concerns about inadequate information about medical procedures and their consequences. The rising number of female physicians, coupled with the growth in nurse-practitioners as primary care providers, has moved women's voices and egalitarian interactional styles closer to the medical mainstream (Eagan, 1994).

For educated women with access to health care choices, the information age has enabled an unprecedented degree of self-determination, self-treatment, and self-advocacy. Women can use computerized searches to locate information about their illnesses, important diagnostic tests, the best forms of treatment, and the most reputable medical centers and physicians. Self-help books abound on ailments ranging from hot flashes to heart disease, and patient education leaflets and videotapes can be seen in almost every physician's office. Pharmaceutical companies now advertise directly to consumers in popular magazines, advising readers to ask their doctors about newer forms of drugs. Many medications once restricted to prescription-only access can be purchased over the counter.

With this explosion of health information in the public domain and a simultaneous surge in research interest in behaviors and traits that increase disease risk comes a new burden on individuals of decision making and responsibility for their own health outcomes. In this new paradigm, illness is viewed in large measure as the fault of the ill person, for not using the latest preventive strategies, not recognizing and acting on symptoms, and not following recommendations for care or denying oneself the indulgences that bring on disease. Individuals now look to their own actions and lifestyles for explanations for illness.

This burden of personal responsibility coexists with a new surge in research on genetic triggers of disease, represented by the Human Genome Project underway at the National Institutes of Health (Lee, 1991). This massive enterprise is designed to map and sequence the entire human genetic code, revealing the sources of inherited diseases and opening the potential for early identification and even genetic treatment of those at risk. So on the one hand, we increasingly believe that the major causes of death, such as AIDS, cancer, and heart disease, are rooted in lifestyle and behavior, and on the other hand we are gathering information about our genetic predispositions, over which we have no control. The consequent confusion in even the most highly-educated health care consumers is predictable.

As caregivers for others as well as themselves, contemporary women carry a heavy charge of knowing the right thing to do for family members who are ill and controlling the family environment and diet to promote health, while at the same time being disadvantaged by lower incomes, multiple role burdens, and social expectations of peacemaking and deference to men. If, as is now widely believed, stress contributes to many illnesses, it is no wonder that women have more doctor visits! At least the likelihood is increasing that their concerns will be heard.

Health Care System Changes

Shrinking public and private financial support for health care has brought dramatic change in the form and content of medical encounters. Health care in the United States is now largely market driven, as the federal government and private insurers have pushed for efficiency through decentralization, privatization, downsizing, and "results budgeting" (Lasker, 1997). Hospital stays are much shorter than 15 years ago and restricted to the most acute phases of illness. No longer is the hospital nurse granted the luxury of time to teach patients about their recovery and be sure they understand or to listen and provide emotional support. In outpatient settings, patients are exposed to receptionists and their busy physicians and rarely have the safety net of professional nurses to monitor their responses to illness. Nurses providing home care may still have the opportunity to listen to patients and families and teach the basic facts about their recent illnesses, the ways their lives will change, and the signs and symptoms of complications. Yet only those with serious illnesses and adequate health insurance receive home care visits.

In increasingly busy outpatient health centers driven by managed care, there is less time overall for teaching and learning, despite increasing burdens on patient and family to perform important aspects of treatment. There is less time for emotional expression and support and less opportunity to correct misdiagnoses and misunderstandings. This is particularly worrisome for patients with language or literacy barriers and for those whose cultural backgrounds include views on health different from the Western biomedical model.

As counselors are well aware, mental health benefits and services have been acutely curtailed by managed care systems to the point where federal legislation has been proposed to ensure a minimal level of mental health coverage. The chronic nature of many mental health problems makes this especially challenging for mental health professionals. With restricted specialist referrals and access, half or more of mental health care and over two thirds of psychotropic medications are now provided or prescribed by general practitioners rather than mental health specialists. This situation continues despite the fact that primary care providers have been found to detect only a small proportion of disorders such as major depression and to be less effective at treating mental illness than are specialists. Brief therapy formats have become the norm rather than a treatment option for selected patients (Mays & Croake, 1997), with results that many mental health providers find less than satisfactory. As women compose the majority of mental health clients, they are especially vulnerable to inadequate treatment.

In this context of ever-briefer contact with health professionals and increasing burden on the individual for self-diagnosis and treatment, self-instruction on the implications of illness, and navigation and negotiation of the complexities of health care, women have little space or time to talk about and process their health and illness experiences. Yet thanks to the women's health movements of the 1970s, many now do value their own perceptions and judgments about their bodies and the causes and treatments of illness. Many women realize they must have the best information and guidance possible to be able to advocate for themselves in increasingly complex health care delivery systems. More than ever, women are in need of informed and compassionate listening and support as they confront the losses and obstacles of illness and recovery.

Loosening of the Biomedical Model

Another recent shift in mainstream biomedicine has been a new respect for and tolerance of alternative and complementary therapies. Acupuncture, herbal treatment, massage and chiropractic, and mind-body approaches, such as relaxation training, visualization, biofeedback, and meditation, are being granted increasing acceptance by medical practitioners. Spiritual healing, long practiced but rarely supported by mainstream medicine, is now receiving increased attention. The women's health movement has supported these alternative approaches as undervalued practices long passed down among women in their caregiver roles. Biomedical practitioners are paying increasing attention to scant but convincing research on the effectiveness of some modalities. Whereas alternative health care methods represent new options for women and often are less costly than physician care, they do require access to information and guidance for women not raised in the ethnic traditions from which these treatments arose.

Alternative healing methods use divergent information sources about health and illness. They promote new understandings of the relationship of health to unity of mind and body and of individual lifestyle to family, environment, and culture. As such, they help validate what women have long espoused, the importance of context, emotions, sense of self, relationships, and harmony with tradition and one's surroundings to women's well-being. Much more information is needed on how these treatments interact with medical therapies and medications. In the meantime, women are struggling to gather relevant information and resources to make challenging health care decisions.

THE IMPORTANCE OF SMALL-SCALE RESEARCH ON WOMEN

In an era of rapid change in the public understanding of the causes of illness, the range of legitimate treatments, the role of patient versus professional, and the importance of including diverse groups and particularly women in health research and planning, counselors are witnessing great complexity and conflict in their clients' lives. Women remain the main consumers of health care and counseling and more than ever need valid information and support in coping with illness. The relative absence of large-scale research on health issues for women requires us to look to other and perhaps richer information sources.

Verbatim accounts from women have great power to convey the experience of illness and suggest avenues for support. In addition, small-scale interview studies are a necessary first step to design larger investigations directed at women's most distressing concerns. Each of these studies is only a tiny window into a few individuals' experiences, but each is designed to facilitate women's explanations of how they view their illnesses in context and what is important to them, rather than what a distant investigator has decided to measure. Although this personal-level research has yet to tap all the diverse groups of U. S. women or study the full range of illness experiences, when the extant findings are grouped and consolidated as in this book, the tiny windows opened by each study combine to form a multifaceted stained glass design that has logical meaning. For counseling purposes, accounts of the experience of illness and recovery can reveal more about potential avenues for therapy than would facts and figures on the prevalence and predictors of disease. With this in mind, we move to a consideration of common pathways through illness and then to the particularities of a variety of illness experiences.

2

Reckoning and Reconciling

A Map of Women's Illness and Recovery

Within women's vividly diverse experiences of illness and trauma, threats to health share a common impact, and the process of adjusting to these hardships has a common core. In this chapter, a road map of the shared characteristics of illness and loss experiences is described. The simple core of the theory portrayed in this chapter is useful as a framework for interpreting clinical observations of women's illness experience and helping women chart a path through what may appear to be insurmountable pain and grief. The forms the framework may take will be explored in much more depth in the chapters that follow, when readers will hear from women experiencing different types of illness and loss situations.

This will be a sometimes somber journey through the world of women's suffering and endurance, a pathway that for some leads over time to brighter and more peaceful ways of life. It is a story of both loss and growth; of external changes in circumstances, relationships, and the body; and internal changes in self-concept and personal future. It involves hard work and waiting, courage and giving up, all of which are parts of coming to terms with illness and finding ways to protect the core of selfhood when everything else has changed.

Counseling suggestions are offered for each task in the process. Familiar techniques of both insight-oriented and cognitive-behavioral therapy can be bolstered by the insights provided in this model of women's pathways through painful life-changing events. The concepts described here certainly are not new to helping professionals. This chapter may simply provide more and different vocabulary for women's tasks of recovery and growth through adversity.

A THEORY OF WOMEN'S ILLNESS EXPERIENCE

Suffering is the emotional experience of physical, emotional, and interpersonal trauma (Morse & Carter, 1995, 1996). Its devastation comes not in the traumatic event but in the realization of its meaning over time. Suffering is painful confrontation with loss of important parts of the self and of links to others and the wider world. *Enduring* often is interspersed with waves of suffering. Enduring is focusing intently on getting through the present when energy and resources are not sufficient to risk being overwhelmed by the distress of suffering (Morse & Carter, 1995, 1996).

TABLE 2.1 Adjustment to Illness and Trauma: Common Threads

Phase	Definition	Tasks
Enduring[a]	Self-protection from suffering by focusing only on present	Survive until resources become available to deal with loss
Suffering[a]	Feeling emotional impact of loss to self in past, present, and future	Experience emotional impact of changes to self, life as it was known, and future that had been taken for granted
Reckoning	Coming to terms with extent of loss	Expand awareness of loss Appraise implications for self See logic of past self
Reconciling	Making peace with changes and integrating into self	Put loss into perspective Take ownership of illness management
Normalizing	Rebuilding life around changed priorities and new sense of self	Shape self-congruent life patterns Work for validating relationships Trust in uncertainty Defend the tender self

[a] SOURCE: Morse & Carter, 1995, 1996.

Across many studies of women's illness experience touched on in this book, we will see that women who survive and grow through suffering use a basic process of *reckoning* and *reconciling*. Reckoning is becoming fully aware of the extent of change brought by illness: facing and coming to terms with the impact of hurt and loss. Reconciling is finding ways to make peace with the change, to reappraise self and situation and put oneself back together again in a new way. The outcome of successful reckoning and reconciling over time is *normalizing*, rejoining life, diminishing the power of illness and hurt, and making a place for the changed self. The components of the process are listed in Table 2.1. Although they are described here as phases or steps in a process, it is important to remember that women cycle in and out of the different parts of the process depending on the issues at hand; the emotional energy available; physical distractions such as pain or fatigue; and many other contextual factors surrounding the adjustment process. They may take a straightforward or roundabout route as they confront the tasks of rebuilding themselves in the face of illness.

SUFFERING: DEMANDS OF ILLNESS AND TRAUMA[1]

Suffering and Enduring

To grasp the depth of the process of reckoning and reconciling, it is essential to appreciate the many forms and aspects of suffering that confront women during illness and trauma. Hurt and threat can be physical, cognitive, or emotional, originating in oneself or in a loved one or relationship. Pain and loss can be in the present, reemerging from the past, or anticipated with dread in the future. Each acute or chronic assault on normal life is a threat to the self, the person one is to oneself and others, including the unique identities we have built, the bodies we move in, skills and roles we have acquired, histories and relationships nurtured, pleasures enjoyed, futures planned--our special fit in the living world.

Suffering is the ordeal of realizing threats, facing them and feeling fear, grief, anger, and emptiness at the prospect of losing the life we have known, the future we had counted on, and the selfhood we have constructed and relied on over time. Suffering is the anguished emotional reality of viewing the impact of loss on the past, present, and future. As Morse and Carter (1995, 1996), veteran researchers of illness experience, concluded after interviewing many persons and families who had experienced severe illness and loss, suffering is intense emotional work that can only be done a bit at a time.

For self-preservation, we intersperse suffering with periods of enduring, defined for our purposes as surviving by blocking distress about past and future and concentrating on the present. Enduring is intently marking time until we have energy or emotional resources to face our changed reality, which brings

---

[1] The author is indebted to Morse and Carter (1996), whose framework for understanding suffering was supported over and over again in the analyses of studies for this book.

suffering again. Enduring is essential to survival; it is not "denial" of the reality of impact of hurt and loss but rather an often conscious choice not to deal with the full meaning of a traumatic event until some later time. Enduring is often the first response to an unthinkable injury or loss. We are unable to grasp, confront, or process it right away; we shut off the flood of sensations and work to get a grip on ourselves until some aid or strength can be gathered. Yet, enduring is hard work in itself and cannot be sustained indefinitely. When we relax our guard, suffering ensues again.

The Many Sources of Suffering

Body Pain

Pain can originate in illness, injury, or as a physical response to emotional trauma: the fear in the pit of the stomach, the lump in the throat, the ache in the heart. It brings fear of damage to our essential relied-upon body, restricts movement, prevents relaxation, and hampers work. It is exhausting, as we steel ourselves against it, push through it, and struggle to endure it by concentrating on other thoughts.

Gender roles affect responses to pain. Women may be particularly vulnerable to suffering when in pain, as often we are not socialized to endure it stoically but instead to be kind to our bodies, not to trust their strength but to recognize their vulnerability, and when in pain to seek comfort and assistance. By the same token, women's claims of pain may be downplayed by others as emotional overreaction or weakness, and their ability to endure it may be doubted by health care providers who either overprescribe pain relievers, when they think strong medicine will be needed as women lack other forms of coping, or underprescribe them, when they think women are exaggerating their claims of pain.

The immobility brought on by chronic pain may contribute to depression. One can feel worthless as a non-participant in life's work, powerless against relentless pain and its theft of the freedom to be spontaneously who we are. Chronic pain threatens relationships, as focusing inward makes it more difficult to focus on the experience of others or nurture them. As pain threatens one's past achievements, present relationships and daily experience, and future dreams, it brings loss of self, which is suffering. Emotional anguish adds to bodily pain.

Body Changes, Visible and Invisible

If we lose a leg or a breast, our bodies are visibly changed. If we lose a uterus or other internal organ surgically, we retain a scar on the skin, but the meaning of the loss of that organ may not be fully apparent to others. Some bodily changes do not create any mark at all, such as the onset of diabetes or leukemia. Yet in all these conditions, women lose the intactness, unity, smooth functioning, and taken-for-grantedness of their bodies as the essential, familiar, valued dwelling places of their selves. Many women feel their bodies reflect their selfhood and their worth.

When Body Functions or Actions are Out of Control

As adults, one of our distinctions from infants and animals is our ability to regulate body functions, such as movement and elimination. We also take for granted that our bodies will not erupt in involuntary acts, such as vomiting, seizures, incontinence, or random movements. These kinds of conditions threaten another part of the self, the self-image as mature, socially appropriate, and in charge of the body. The Western notion of the mind as controlling the body by intellect, training, and will is deeply embedded in everyday social consciousness, and women whose illnesses limit this control face stigma and self-disappointment, even when they know the biomedical reason for their loss of control.

Being Contagious

For women with HIV or herpes, for example, having a body that can harm others simply by contact brings suffering. When touch cannot be offered out of love or compassion and when sexual intimacy becomes cruelty instead of a gift of pleasure and caring, women lose not only their bodies as tools of sharing and nurturing but themselves as good and beneficent. We become alienated from others and doubt our worth. Furthermore, the presumed source of our infections in careless or promiscuous sexual contact casts further aspersions on our self-control.

Losing Ability, Mobility, and Spontaneity

Many chronic diseases and traumatic damage, such as arthritis, multiple sclerosis, or spinal cord injury, limit women's ability to perform physical tasks, to move independently, and to act spontaneously without compensating for illness or risk. One of the hardest blows of loss of ability and mobility is becoming dependent and requiring assistance from others, often the family members for whom a woman would have provided care if she were able. In addition to being a burden on others, one loses agency, the capacity to do what one wants and needs to do to maintain roles and identities. The mind struggles and the body says no.

Lacking Energy to Be Oneself

Fatigue is a component of many illnesses and is a frustrating and depressing restriction on agency and self-renewal. Without energy, the powerlessness and hopelessness of depression is close behind, and depression further saps women's capacities and confidence for moving and doing. In a society where worth is often measured in accomplishment and meeting one's responsibilities, persistent overwhelming fatigue can lead to a feeling of worthlessness.

Living in an Uncertain, Unpredictable Body

Some diseases bring with them extreme fluctuations from day to day and season to season. Uncertainty is a powerful stressor in many illness situations; it throws all the assumed events and achievements of the future into question. Women wonder, Will I be well enough to work? Will I live to see my grandchild born? Will my arthritis be so painful that I must spend the day in bed instead of celebrating my birthday with loved ones? An unpredictable body robs one of the unconscious, taken-for-granted ease of moving through the world, influencing situations, participating in the eventual rewards of labor, and helping others and replaces it with worry, the shame of dependency, and fear.

Emotional Pain: Bitter Losses

Suffering and negative health consequences can be rooted in interpersonal harm and loss. For example, some women's eating disorders or alcoholism may be means of coping with the pain of past sexual abuse or ongoing domestic violence. Women who suffered harm as young children carry a damaged sense of self into adulthood and with it, uncertainty about basic values, appropriate behavior, and safety in daily life. Their stories detail the most acute and pervasive suffering of all women's health conditions examined for this book, in that the harms they suffered deprived them of both comfort and security in life and the tools by which to manage their present situations and obtain help. Their efforts to relieve suffering are often harmfully self-directed, as the self is the very source of pain.

Living in a Dying Body

Women who are aware that they face death suffer in commonly understood ways and also in ways few have discussed. As we consider our deaths, the ultimate loss of selfhood, we may grieve for achievements left undone, obligations unfulfilled, satisfactions denied us, and losses to our children and other loved ones without our presence and nurturing. We also may grieve for loss of the living body, rage against diseases that have stolen our health and capacity for living, and feel isolated and powerless as strength and function slip away. This hurt may be magnified by the suffering of being unable to find meaning or purpose in all the successive losses. Who am I, and what am I worth, if my life is being taken so soon? How can I give and grow as I had planned? How does my death fit into the universe I thought I had understood?

What Suffering Means: Threats to an Integrated Self

This catalog of suffering serves to remind us of how our bodies carry our selfhood and our future. When our bodies are threatened, suffering results. Yet as Morse and Carter (1996) observed, and not unfeelingly, to suffer is the first step toward working through loss and reformulating a different self. We are familiar with advice to the bereaved to express their grief so they can move on. A similar process happens in serious illness, when the anguish of coming face to face with physical and emotional pain and its implications for one's future is the necessary beginning of the next struggle, of reckoning with it.

Counseling Women Who Are Suffering

The Protective Value of Enduring

Women encountered in the early stages of illness may be either suffering or enduring. Enduring is self-protection for survival of the physical body, the integrity of the self, or both (Morse & Carter, 1995). The fierce concentration of simply getting through the present, whether a hospitalization for cancer treatment, the initial days after the death of a loved one, or an exacerbation of the pain of arthritis, will require conscious or unconscious denial of the wider implications of the events. Women may refuse counseling intervention at this point if they perceive it as extra work or obligation or if they sense they do not have the strength to examine their situations any more closely than necessary to endure them. Those who do accept professional psychological help may be looking for concrete facts about their physical problems to help them minimize the threats, rather than for emotional release and support. Yet a counseling presence is an important resource for later, when suffering breaks through. When is enduring appropriate, and when does it constitute unhealthy denial? Many authors agree that denial is basically a healthy self-protection and indicates that a woman does not yet have the inner resources to deal with the threats imposed by illness (Lubkin, 1995, p. 248). The counselor's task is to identify and bolster strengths and coping strategies so that the threat gradually becomes manageable, starting with emotional support and validation and then perhaps later, if denial becomes a health threat, using cognitive interventions to gently challenge distorted thinking.

Counselors must be careful not to agree with patently false hopes and beliefs. This is a difficult tightrope to walk. Two avenues may be helpful: First, focus on what the woman has accepted about the illness and shore up strategies for dealing with that part of the loss. When that part becomes manageable, other aspects of the loss can be taken on in turn. Second, using speculation or fictitious case studies, present similar illness situations and help the woman to identify the threat that would underlie the illness if her case were indeed that severe. This is a bit more gentle than the worst-case scenario, which is overtly personal. Over time, examining the rational and irrational fears associated with that threat can make the illness easier to reckon with. Sadly, it may take an acute exacerbation of illness, as in the alcoholic's "hitting bottom," to demonstrate to some women that they must reckon with their loss.

Meanwhile, critically important self-care and treatment may be missed, and the woman's health may decline further. Here, the counselor needs to work with reference materials and other health professionals to learn about the health problem, find out the important signs of deterioration, and gain understanding of the purpose and importance of various treatments to portray to the woman the consequences of not participating and work with her to identify symptoms of worsening disease. Becoming well-informed about a client's illness condition will also help counselors distinguish the reactions and psychological changes that are linked to the illness from those that may predate the physical health problem.

In acute episodes, it may be appropriate to enhance strategies for enduring, rather than attempting to elicit suffering. Nurses' coaching of women through childbirth is one example of this intervention. These strategies may include distraction techniques and other activities such as counting, visualization, relaxation, mental focusing on something of value, or dividing time into manageable blocks, whether minutes, hours, or days. For a temporary condition such as a painful medical procedure, suffering may be staved off until the threat has passed, but women whose losses will be sustained into the future must eventually let the awareness of loss flood in.

Facilitating Suffering

Suffering will erupt when there are inner and outer resources to begin to face the reality of the threat (Morse & Carter, 1996). Women must feel some degree of strength or protection from other threats before they can allow themselves to really suffer--to risk being overwhelmed by the grief and fear of the present illness. Counselors can provide important external support to enable women to let go of the fatiguing strategy of enduring and delve into suffering. They may simply offer a therapeutic presence and empathetic listening during suffering, normalizing the extreme emotional and physical responses of active grief and encouraging significant others to do the same. They may also become actively involved in reality testing with the woman to verify the nature of the threat and the meaning of the pain.

Not only do illnesses vary in their threats to the self, but women's personal values and histories impose unique meaning on their individual experiences of illness and loss. For one woman, the diagnosis of heart disease may mean needing to accept personal vulnerability and the need for daily medication. For another it may mean prophecies of inherited risk and early death fulfilled, concern about young children's health and nurturing in the future, loss of income from a strenuous blue-collar job, and so forth. Illness acuity and severity vary from woman to woman, and the impact is personalized in ways counselors may not begin to understand until the difficult process of reckoning begins.

Although a few may prefer to suffer alone, many women's need during suffering is acute: for supportive others, for awareness that an end is possible, for understanding that whatever can be done is being done. Counselors may coach family members to offer reassurance. This can be most effective when families are helped to understand that the woman's needs at the moment are basic, not heroic--companionship, touch, listening, reassurance, food and rest--yet critical to preserving enough selfhood to move on and integrate the loss.

RECKONING: MEASURING THE MAGNITUDE OF LOSS

Probing the Extent of Hurt and Threat

The task of reckoning is sizing up and accepting what is left after the onslaught of trauma or illness. As counselors have long understood, this is more easily said than done. Women diagnosed with multiple sclerosis, heart disease, or diabetes may initially be distracted by the many practical tasks of diagnosis and treatment or may feel secure in the medical plans to control their illness and only later confront the real impact of the affliction on their lives. Meanwhile, over time illness may continue to bring more losses, unforeseen situations may reveal new obstacles, and reckoning must occur over and over again.

Counselors can recognize women's efforts at reckoning in women's stories of how life has changed and how little of the old normality remains. This awareness may come freely as illness is experienced over time, or it may come only with counseling work if it has been too threatening to encounter without help. As in bereavement (Edelstein, 1994), reckoning is holding on while letting go, struggling to preserve something of value while facing the meaning of the change that has occurred.

Tools for Enhancing Awareness and Appraisal

Awareness is a cognitive process, facing the here and now. Appraisal is a self-examination process, judging the impact of what is here now. They can be facilitated by insight-oriented therapy and introspection, by cognitive strategies of reality testing, and by peer encounters that demonstrate to women how their illnesses can be viewed as manageable and incorporated into living. Yet awareness and appraisal cannot be rushed through, even for women with a great deal of insight and expert help. The meaning of illness is only revealed over time, as daily events and periodic milestones bring to awareness how life has changed and how illness or trauma affects one's personal landscape.

For example, women with cancer may at first be so busy with surgery and starting chemotherapy and so invested in the plan of treatment that they see themselves in medical terms, as a case with certain odds for survival or cure. Over time, they have a different experience, as they cope with the repeated shock of seeing themselves in mirrors or the disheartening failures of the afflicted body to do what it has always so easily done. They find that fatigue catches them unaware and that they cannot count on being able to drive or eat or sleep well. Thus, the impact of cancer and its treatment on their daily lives and their future becomes real only over time.

As women begin honest self-appraisal, they let go of illusions of normality, of being able to go about their business. They begin to look at how the loss affects their sense of who they are. In doing so, they forgive themselves for their own failures to make the illness go away or become unimportant. They take stock of their own weakness and need and of their strength and resourcefulness. They give up the illusion of successful management of chronic illness with short-term fixes and begin the search for long-term strategies. The longevity of the loss sets in. But in seeing clearly the extent of their losses, women also can begin to grasp what remains. They take stock of the resources they have left, the abilities that endure despite incapacity. Simply having survived the loss clinging to some shred of selfhood can be seen as proof of possibility and hope. They view loved ones and significant supporters with new eyes and accept the possibility of being able to use the available help. Priorities begin to shift.

Counselors can facilitate this inventory taking, nudging gently to help women catalog both what is lost and what remains. Just as the alcoholic must come to grips over time with her continuing compulsion to drink and the underlying pain that prompts it, the woman who has heart disease must see how her daily routine will be changed by the need to attend to diet, medications, activity levels, and symptoms. Events of daily living bring these matters into view, and counselors can help women process through each as it emerges. Diary assignments or review of a typical day can provide the opening for discussion of illness' impact on daily life and future expectations.

Medical information is important to many women who are working on coming to terms with chronic illness. Women may seek out hospital libraries or research journals to find full and accurate information about little-known conditions. Health professionals and counselors can help women and inform themselves by locating and providing clients with literature that is current and complete without being patronizing or overly simplistic. Women can be helped to interpret medical literature so as not to place undue emphasis on single research studies or recent media reports.

Women who feel they have the informational tools to judge for themselves what is known about their illnesses will be empowered to participate in their own treatment. Furthermore, understanding the biomedical origins of an illness can help to correct women's misconceptions and ease guilt or shame about their own roles in bringing it on or making it worse. Counselors who are well-informed about their clients' diseases and treatments will be better able to help them distinguish the losses that were indeed preventable from those that were beyond voluntary control.

Seeing the Logic of the Past Self

When illness causes a woman to see herself in new light, she may acquaint herself differently with the woman she has been. Women beginning to work on eating disorders or substance abuse problems move beyond facile explanations of their compulsion to a deeper understanding of how their behaviors have been keeping them intact. Such realizations can bring terror, as they pull the fabric of coping from a woman who feels she was barely managing as it was. Women with heart disease may look back and realize they had explained away their long-term symptoms based on conventional beliefs that heart disease is a man's problem and that chest pain is the usual sign of trouble. They may see how they had pushed their symptoms aside in favor of responding to other priorities, such as job tasks or care of children and family. Many may see more clearly the failings of health professionals and others in whom they had placed their faith. As women review and come to understand their present illnesses, they also gain new knowledge of their past selves and reckon with their own and others' weaknesses and strengths.

Counseling Challenges in Reckoning

Downward Comparison as Comfort

A common strategy women use to measure the impact of loss is minimization or downward comparison. When women frame their losses as not as bad as they could be or not as bad as others' predicaments, counselors usually will be most helpful by supporting this coping strategy rather than scrutinizing it. When women are clearly aware of the extent of their changed circumstances, minimization is not denial; rather, it is a way of placing one's losses in context along the continuum of possible tragedy. This is a healthy sign and is part of reaffirming what one has left to work with.

Can counselors point out those "worse off," to help women gain this perspective and hope? If the comparison acknowledges the magnitude of loss and doesn't falsely belittle its impact, it may be helpful. Otherwise, when a woman is immersed in mourning a loss, any message that "it's not so bad" it may be perceived as an affront. Minimization must come from within or be endorsed fully by the woman before it can be built on as a source of strength.

Support Through Ups and Downs

Women need to know that the adjustment process of reckoning with illness and trauma may be interspersed with periods of acute grief and of grim enduring. This waxing and waning occurs in response to evolving internal insight and external context. For example, a new realization of the meaning of loss may prompt a new bout of grieving, as when chronic illness takes a downward turn or a woman is confronted for the first time with a task she formerly performed that she now cannot do. Counselors can support women to see that the reckoning process continues in new ways over time. Even when the basic fact of a loss has been accepted, its meaning evolves as each new situation reveals new aspects of the loss.

Grief or Depression?

Reckoning can bring depression when women see what is lost but cannot yet see what remains for them. Untreated depression in women with physical illness may lead to increased illness severity and loss of life (Davis & Jensen,

1988). Conventional depression treatment is important, including medication; cognitive reframing of excessively negative self-portraits; behavioral structuring of daily activities to reduce a sense of uselessness or powerlessness; insight-oriented therapy focused on the biographical work of rethinking past, present, and future; and social interventions to reduce withdrawal and boost self-esteem.

Medications for depression must be carefully chosen and doses calculated with medical consultation about an ill woman's digestive, liver, and kidney function, to avoid overdose or exacerbation of physical problems of illness. Counselors who prescribe or refer a woman for psychotropic drugs should be sure that the prescriber is aware of the woman's physical condition and her other medications. At the same time, it is important not to shy away from antidepressant medications only for fear of interfering with medical treatments. Improving her daily quality of life may enable a woman to participate better in the plan of care as well as move forward in the adjustment process.

Women facing severe illness may resist a diagnosis of depression. They may see this label as implying that their grief is inappropriate or their troubles are all in their heads. They must be supported in their accurate perceptions of loss and encouraged to vent their grief, anger, and frustration. Psychotherapeutic interventions can be framed in terms of finding ways to live with the illness and not as cure for depression alone. Feelings of sadness and incapacitating grief and emptiness must be carefully explored to distinguish important mourning of losses from prolonged interference with daily functioning.

Counselors who build productive relationships with women are well positioned to recognize whether the important internal work of reckoning is going on or whether a woman is stuck in depression and needs additional resources or intervention to move forward. Professional helpers play important roles in emotional support, reality testing, problem-solving, and family involvement as women reckon with their unique illness situations.

When Loss is Not Reckoned With

Women who are unable to discover or come to terms with the changes they face are detoured or caught up in lacunae of continued suffering. Those who cannot see any strength or hope remaining after they face the enormity of their weakness and loss may dwindle into depression. Those who feel too weak or lack the skills to encounter and experience the pain of their losses may subdue the pain by misguided problem solving, such as self-harm, substance abuse, or bulimia. Those who see no easy way to fit the demands of a disease into their lives may continue to ignore it until a health crisis occurs. Those who have not yet internalized the reality of their difference from those unaffected by illness, such as women with diabetes or overweight who struggle to adhere to a diet plan while craving the comfort and normalcy of spontaneous, unregulated eating, may find themselves in cycles of "frustration-cheat-repent" (Armstrong, 1990). This may be the state of affairs when a woman seeks help in counseling. By recognizing the work that hasn't yet been done to reckon with the changes brought by illness and using simple tools and support, counselors can help women move forward in the process. Yet rarely is recovery a straight line. To reckon with illness and loss, many women cycle painfully back and forth between fighting their differences and the sacrifices they entail and working to accept losses and make something of what remains.

RECONCILING:
GAINING PERSPECTIVE, TAKING OWNERSHIP

Putting Loss into Perspective

Reconciling is making peace with illness and change and reclaiming the individuality and self-direction that is part of one's sense of self. It may begin by reconnecting with the body. Once women have begun to look unflinchingly at what has befallen them, they can begin to own and find love for this changed "me." Rather than looking in the mirror and seeing "me missing my breast," the woman sees "me in my body now." Likewise, a woman recovering from an unexpected heart attack may accept explanations for the event and the limitations she will face henceforth, but she must also make part of herself the actual differences in how she feels from day to day and integrate her healing heart into who she is: her relationships, priorities and routines.

Introspection facilitated by journal keeping, therapeutic discussion, and validation from others is critical to this effort. Counselors can help women move from seeing only a missing breast when they look in the mirror to seeing the whole body with its remaining capacity for beauty and good and the sparks of selfhood that shine in the eyes. Body mapping, self-portraits in words or other media, and physical reconnection with the body are all useful. Perhaps most valuable are others' affirmations of the woman's continued importance, uniqueness, and capacity to give, as well as others' enduring love for her. Counselors can facilitate this communication in families and relationships.

Reconnecting with the body is a physical experiential process as well. Massage can help a woman connect with the form and sensation of her body, and relaxation techniques and visualization can bring women back to experience of the body as whole. To the extent possible, getting out and doing physical activities, even ones that seem at first like pleasureless ordeals, can bring women a sense of what strength and capacity remain to them. Intimate relationships become an important arena for women's reconciling with their bodies. Given many women's cultural burden of proving their worth through their appearance, being accepted in a less-than-perfect body becomes part of self-acceptance and self-love. Personal growth also can occur as women identify their abilities and assets beyond the physical. Counseling sensitivity, coaching to enhance communication and creative thinking in intimate relationships, and support for women taking these brave steps can be crucial.

Peer support is extremely helpful in reconciling with a changed body. Whether through groups for those with a similar illness or by one-on-one connections with others living with the same condition, women can come to see how others create self-directed lives despite illness. Peer support also helps women reconnect with their individuality beyond the illness. In a group of others who share something that would otherwise separate them from "normal" society, the difference is no longer a difference, and the personhood of group members can be appreciated. Role modeling can occur, and feedback from the group reminds women of their own unique srengths and qualities. Practical skills for dealing with illness-related problems can also be shared. Just as Alcoholics Anonymous has developed a folklore of cognitive-behavioral self-help tips (living "one day at a time," recognizing self-destructive "stinking thinking"), other illness-specific groups share ways of coping and practical strategies for managing disability, pain, work and family issues, and treatment difficulties.

Women in areas where such groups are unavailable may go to great lengths on their own to connect with others like themselves, by corresponding with national groups or even by starting groups of their own. Books and media resources are also very important in reconciling. Counselors can direct women to literature such as the works referred to later in this book that go beyond medical descriptions of disease to describe the inner experience of women coping with illness. As they work toward reconciling with illness, women want evidence that it can be done: concrete examples of others who have figured out how to respond to a particular disease and still lead a meaningful life. They also seek to reduce the feeling of aloneness that emerged in the reckoning phase, when they saw how the meaning and demands of illness set them apart from family and friends.

Making Sense of the Body's Breakdown

Reconciling also entails developing a logical understanding of the illness in the flow and context of the way life was and where it is going. This exploration can be medical, practical, relational, and spiritual. At times, women focus on understanding the medical reasons why this illness occurred, to integrate this vulnerability into their self-concepts and future plans. Sometimes, this information is available, and at other times, there is no complete biomedical explanation for what happened. In the case of unexplained illness or traumatic injury or loss, women work on the existential question of "why me?" seeking a way to make peace with the massive intrusion into their responsible lives, their lack of control over such threats, and their inability to protect others from similar events. The journey can be difficult and stormy before a new logic or understanding emerges. Some women accomplish this peacemaking by finding greater appreciation of life and gratitude for survival and by more assertively expressing their appreciation of others. Spiritual and religious explanations are also important.

Counselors can encourage women to communicate their developing understanding of the reasons for illness and work on a culturally congruent explanation that maximizes the potential for improvement. This may mean in-depth discussion of the medical knowledge base; exploration of various psychological and behavioral theories about complex problems, such as addiction and eating disorders; trying on alternative explanations offered by non-Western approaches, such as traditional Chinese medicine or yoga; or developing personal models of explanation from within their own life experience.

Counselors can explore women's religious beliefs and practices optimize the support and explanatory power these resources can offer. At the same time, serious illness can bring women to question their prior religious assumptions and faith. Counselors may need to examine with women the way their religious doctrines can be reinterpreted or reframed to help make sense of life events. If this revisioning is beyond the range of their original spiritual tradition, some women begin to explore other avenues of belief and spiritual comfort.

Owning the Illness: Taking Control Back

Making Choices to Sustain the Self

In reconciling, the illness becomes part of the self. The focus of work goes beyond illness management to expanding the boundaries of selfhood to rise above it. This can require taking chances and pushing past old limits. For example, as women with arthritis accept their increasing limitations, they also may begin to test the limits of their mobility and persevere though pain to rejoin the activities that matter to them. Those suffering from abuse by a domestic partner may come to decide that although the pain and risk of leaving home is tremendous, reclaiming their integrity is worth it. Facing a recurrence of cancer, a woman comes to realize that this is indeed her very own life and her death, and only she can decide how to spend her remaining months. An existential awareness of both aloneness and choice accompanies women's taking charge of illness.

Not Fitting the Medical Model

As women gain experience in living with illness conditions, they often find that their bodily responses do not follow exactly the patterns described by health professionals. Recommended therapies may not work to relieve pain, improve mobility, stabilize blood sugar, or lighten mood or may not be worth the trouble. One of the hardest blows is finding that health professionals really do not know enough about an illness condition to help beyond the initial diagnostic period and that a woman is on her own to find manageable and effective self-care practices. This brings both burden and empowerment. Women work to become reconciled to their responsibilities for self-determination in the face of illness. They take charge of shaping their perhaps diminished but personally orchestrated future. They come to see, "No one but me can do this for me." Women may gradually begin tailoring their own care, taking liberties with medication use, abandoning prescribed therapies in favor of other self-designed measures, or seeking additional information from others with the condition or from libraries and news sources. They realize that they now know more about their unique condition than do the professionals, and they judge medical advice against their own predictions of its effect.

Cultural, educational, social, religious, and family contexts all influence women's views of their power to shape the course of illness and the choices available to them. Women without postsecondary education may not have encountered concepts of biology and psychology or may not follow current events or medical news. If a woman's religion teaches submission to the will of God and her culture expects obedience to her husband, her version of taking control of illness will be different from that of the woman who has been raised to believe that she has the capacity to achieve a high level of wellness and the responsibility to participate in decisions regarding her care.

Counselors accustomed to a partnership model of health care in which the client is autonomous must listen especially carefully for a woman's expectations that the doctor, head of the family, or leader of her religious group will make health care decisions. Sensitivity, creativity, and insight in counseling will be needed to bridge cultural and social differences and discover a level of self-determination that is congruent with a woman's background to the degree she desires yet maximizes her quality of life. Sometimes, a woman breaks with her background or religious tradition to pursue what seems like the most healthy course of action during illness. She then faces decisions about how much to reconnect as time goes on. Unspoken assumptions about social roles, such as mother, daughter, or worker, or about health, illness, or life itself can be revealed and perhaps challenged in new ways through counseling.

Supporting Treatment Choices

Owning illness management means seeing the options for treatment and thoughtfully choosing in congruence with one's sense of self and one's view of the world. Women may make an existential choice not to participate in medical treatment for terminal illness, if their understanding is that illness is part of God's plan or that treatment will have no advantage and may cause more pain to loved ones than simply allowing illness to run its course. On the other hand, some women may perceive that they must try all possible attempts at cure to feel satisfied with their own participation or to meet their responsibility to their families. Helpers are challenged to enter into a woman's own worldview and visualize the choices open to her within that life-world. Counseling may influence a woman's awareness of information about her illness and possible treatments, but her ongoing participation in that care will depend on its congruence with her unique priorities.

On good days and bad days, the meaning of illness can shift back and forth from punishment or bad luck to opportunity or challenge (Charmaz, 1991). Women's abilities to be present to and work with their changing bodies may shift, depending on the amount of physical distress they feel on a given day and the contexts of their limitations. Their sense of control may wax and wane depending on the daily success of their strategies to manage illness and its limitations. Yet the ups and downs of reconciling to illness bring women lasting strength and self-respect. As the self successfully integrates the revisions imposed by illness, it grows increasingly able to accept other changes as life goes on. Reconciling may never be fully completed, but many women can experience growth and achieve psychological comfort as they gain perspective on their illnesses and ownership of its demands.

Difficulties in Reconciling

Women with severely limiting and painful chronic illness may have periods of waxing and waning reconciliation. Some days may be more hopeful and peaceful, whereas other days may be difficult to endure. The greater the portion of time spent in a state of reconciliation, the less will be a woman's stress and depression, and the more likely she will be to work with the illness rather than against it.

Although ups and downs are expected, instead of eventually reconciling with illness some women continue to struggle against it, fighting its restrictions and assaults, feeling unjustly harmed. Women who are unaware of others who have achieved satisfactory long-term survival of illness, who lack a sense of self as enduring and resourceful or experience of success in other areas of life, or who had been without support and validation before the advent of their new flaws have fewer cognitive tools to use in reconciling. Larger losses may take more time to reconcile. Cultural patterns of understanding and living with illness affect the ease with which women adjust. For example, those in a cultural context where illness is perceived as an expected part of life or as God's will may reconcile with it sooner than would a woman who sees her illness as a product of her own weakness or a controllable malfunction.

In the absence of reconciliation, illness is a burden and an affront to the self rather than a part of the self. Women faced with this burden without hope of relief may wonder whether life is worth living. Resentment and smoldering anger at the self and others may lead to social isolation, antisocial behavior, depression, suicidality, worsening illness, and death.

NORMALIZING: FINDING A BALANCED LIFE

Shaping a Self-Congruent Pattern

Reconciliation with illness enables women to develop lifestyles that suit the needs and priorities of the newly integrated self. Making almost normal a major blow to health and selfhood, creating daily patterns that reduce it to a less-than-central role and allow other priorities to dominate, may seem preposterous or impossible at first. The tasks of normalizing include submitting to monitoring and self-regulation amidst the flow of illness, making peace with uncertainty, developing validating relationships, and finding voice to advocate for self. As these are basic skills of productive adulthood, counselors are familiar with ways of enhancing them. Normalizing trauma or chronic illness requires better-than-average psychological adjustment. Illness may bring troublesome areas to light that women had formerly been able to ignore, and it may require using old identities and self-management skills in new ways.

Reconciliation with illness brings increased awareness of one's uniqueness, strengths, and life priorities. It motivates women to make a place among their other routines and responsibilities for illness care and its limitations. Simultaneously, it spurs women to restructure their goals to include what now seems important in the new context of illness. They may let go of former pastimes and expectations that no longer fit with the reintegrated self. Over time, life with illness becomes normal life. Illness can at times fade into the background, even as women take the daily steps and make the many concessions necessary to meet its demands.

Negotiating the Tasks of Illness

Many illnesses, including diabetes, arthritis, heart disease, cancer and its treatment, and chronic pain conditions, often require complex self-monitoring and self-care, along with frequent consultation with health professionals. Periods of exacerbation must be anticipated and endured. Medications and their effects must be tracked. For employed women, taking care of their illness needs must be squeezed into the work day. Those with young children or who care for other ill or aged family members must care for themselves while responding to the demands of others. Financial concerns mount with the costs of illness care and women's lost income. Women struggle to maintain equanimity and productivity in the face of many restrictions on movement and social interaction. They may be denied the pleasure of eating and drinking as they would like. The unstructured comfort of leisure time may be absorbed by illness procedures, hampered by fatigue, or made dreary by social isolation.

Monitoring their illness course and their success at managing illness becomes second nature to women as they normalize illness. Each day, many subtle changes are tracked and compensated for. Women become skilled at watching the flow of the effects of illness, at tuning into the body and believing its messages. Some forms of monitoring are in the hands of health professionals, and women with prolonged illness learn to fit medical tests and fear of bad results into their other concerns and priorities. Women who successfully work their way beyond substance abuse or other health behavior problems become adept at monitoring their outlook and thinking processes and taking remedial action when they find self-destructive patterns reemerging. Women develop new respect for bodily sensations and emotions as messages about the self's well-being.

Women negotiate the parts of self-care and self-regulation that are essential for their desired level of health, the steps that will optimize well-being but are perhaps expendable in the face of other priorities, and the procedures and advice that may be helpful to others but do not fit into their own personalized illness experiences and life contexts. Some must be helped to let go of the myth that spontaneity and unlimited indulgence represent normalcy and find other ways of self-nurturing and self-reward. Counselors can support women's work on self-regulation with insight-oriented therapy to explore the meanings of effortless spontaneity. Cognitive restructuring can modify exaggerated thinking about how much freedom has actually been lost.

Self-regulation may require finding out what really happens when one disregards treatment recommendations or medical advice. The seriousness of the medical condition and the importance of choosing to adhere to the regime become very real. As this cold truth becomes accepted, women must work toward making place for illness demands in their identities and lives. This is a most difficult integration process and often involves moments of distress, especially in early months. Counselors can help women avert serious lapses in self-care by teaching them to recognize signs of frustration, make contact with feelings of hopelessness, and take action to get support or relieve stress.

Women who by culture and personal history are accustomed to focusing on others' needs and tolerating their own symptoms without complaining may drop out of rehabilitation programs when they have regained enough strength to go back to caring for home and family (Hawthorne, 1993). In contrast, women for whom a high level of health has been taken for granted may feel more compelled to participate in rehabilitation programs, counseling, and opportunities to rework themselves and their lives (Fleury, Kimbrell, & Kruszewski, 1995). Those with prior illness experience or who are older may have developed coping strategies that can be applied to the new problem or may accept bothersome symptoms more readily than a young women for whom the same illness represents a major threat. The younger woman may spend more time consulting health professionals and trying various remedies to regain the maximal level of comfort and activity (Charmaz, 1995; King & Jensen, 1994). The greater the desire for spontaneity, freedom from restriction, and freedom from an "ill" identity, the less likely is a woman to acquiesce to the demands of illness care.

Dealing with Health Care Systems

Health professionals influence women's self-care patterns by the information they provide and the goals they set for patients. Health care delivery systems often present serious barriers to women seeking personalized or attentive care. The complexities of health care interactions are beyond the scope of this book (see Thorne, 1993, for a closer look), but several points are important in counseling.

Doctors and nurses dispense their stores of information and skill based on judgments about what will work for a patient and what the woman's priorities should be. Their medical care and health teaching is tailored to their understanding of illness and their experience with large numbers of patients, but unless a therapeutic relationship with a patient has revealed her uniqueness over time, care may not be matched to the unique views and circumstances of an individual woman. A health professional may provide detailed information to a woman who seems intelligent and motivated and not give the information to another woman who is judged to be unable or unmotivated to learn details about her illness or follow a strict regime.

Ethnic and cultural differences, ageism, sexism, ableism, and other stereotypes of people's limitations affect health care providers' judgments about what their patients want and need. Likewise, based on their own education, experience, and circumstances, women may or may not go beyond the information provided by their doctors to seek out other sources of insight about their diseases or other ways of treating them. As financial support and options for health care shrink in the face of managed care and capitation systems, even highly motivated women face obstacles in their attempts to obtain the kinds of care that fit their self-concepts and life contexts. They may develop "constructive noncompliance," not fully following medical advice for logical self-protective reasons (Thorne, 1990), which may be appropriate and healthier in the long run. Women whose cultural milieu has fostered dependence and acceptance of limits placed by authority will need guidance, support, and advocacy to define their health care needs and find that care.

Working for Validating Relationships

As women often understand themselves and set priorities based on relationships, ties with significant others must adjust as women normalize their lives around illness. At the onset of illness, many women's first thoughts are for their loved ones and their responsibilities to them. Illness may be denied or not dealt with when caring for others prevents seeking attention for one's own symptoms. Finding ways to meet responsibilities to others during illness is foremost in many women's minds. The support of a partner, friends, or family may sustain a woman through frightening and painful ordeals until she can find her own strength again, and the validation of others may be the main source of self-worth for women during early recovery from life-changing illness or trauma.

Relationship patterns often must be adjusted as women come to understand themselves differently and learn the demands of illness care. Women may need to relinquish roles and responsibilities, receive care from those whom they had previously cared for, or set limits on their involvement or contribution to the lives of others. Family, friends, and employers may need to adjust their perceptions of the woman who is changing her ways of living and interacting in response to illness.

Relationships also shape women's abilities to normalize illness and loss. The available support and help with self-care and her responsibilities to others can determine the degree to which a woman is able to fulfill illness and treatment demands. The level of trust and confidence a woman places in those who take over her responsibilities may make the difference between illness as a manageable part of self or an impossibility given her other duties. Stress due to conflicted relationships or loneliness can lead to loss of confidence and motivation to take proper care of oneself.

Developing validating relationships in and outside of therapy is a primary area for counseling work. A woman facing illness and loss often can benefit from reexamination of her relationship networks and patterns. The importance of others in her sense of who she is and the limits of what others can provide are fruitful areas to explore. How much am I on my own with this cancer pain, and how much can others help? Who will be there for me now that I have lost my sight or my foot to diabetes? What should my children know about our future together now that I have HIV? Why is it so hard to ask my husband for help? Will he think less of me if I don't cook for him or make love as often? How can people love me when I still am struggling to love my changed self? Relationships are the vehicle by which many women will persevere in times of self-doubt. To gain this support, they may need to role-play asking for help and accepting or refusing help. The therapeutic alliance can be an arena for insight and skill building toward healthy and equitable relationships.

Trusting in an Uncertain Future

Both acute and chronic illness bring a new awareness of the uncertainty of life. One of the major tasks of normalizing illness is finding a way to tolerate living with uncertainty and trust that oneself and others can adjust over time to future unknowns. Women learn by experience of survival and adaptation that they can trust in their inner strengths and resourcefulness. Confidence levels may wax and wane with the ebb and flow of illness and its effects, but women reconciled to illness are able to find reassurance that they will be able to handle what comes next. They come to trust their bodies more deeply, even as the bodies surprise them with new forms and manifestations of illness. Learning to live with a changing and self-determining body enables women to understand more deeply how their selves are indeed embodied and to feel acceptance and gratitude for their imperfect bodies.

Trust in others is enhanced when women are able to repattern relationships to meet their newer needs to receive care as well as to give care and make contributions to others' lives. It may take months or years, but to know that others will persist with them through illness, that family can survive without women holding full responsibility for nurturing, and that professionals such as counselors and health workers are available resources in times of need will smooth women's paths toward normalizing illness.

For many women, trust takes on a spiritual dimension. Women who come to believe that whatever happens in the uncertain future is under the care of a supreme Other or a larger design may find confidence that, with this help, they will find strength to continue. Rituals of belief and faith can bring comfort, and inner questioning about "why this illness, why me, why have I lost my taken-for-granted future?" may be resolved with either spontaneous or deliberate reconnection with spiritual life.

As counselors persevere in helping relationships over time and reaffirm women's intactness and survival through illness and loss, women can be helped to gain belief in their own resilience and resourcefulness and encouraged to see these as tools for coping with future events. Professionals can establish solid, open therapeutic relationships that will be available to return to as women move out on their own. Periodically reviewing their supports and strategies for help-seeking will keep these tools for coping ready to hand.

Defending the Tender Self

To sustain new patterns of living and relating, women begin to advocate for their needs in new ways. Even as they become more attuned to their vulnerabilities and the uncertainty of future events, they are compelled to defend their perhaps fragile boundaries. To preserve their energy and focus for their newly affirmed healing priorities, women become more adept at saying no to demands or invitations, challenging unreasonable expectations of others, defending their choices of reduced work involvement, and other instances of preserving resources for healing. Sometimes, a woman defends herself from treatment and compliance demands of health care providers, such as refusing unnecessary tests or appointments, based on her own understanding of what she needs to sustain meaningful life.

For some women, speaking out seems second nature. Counselors will encounter women who are very vocal and assertive from the start in planning illness treatment and obtaining information and help. Although assertiveness initially may compensate for powerlessness in the face of illness, fears and grief may emerge later and with great intensity. For women who have been confident in their own worth and abilities and successful in managing many complex life situations, illness may bring the first serious loss of control. The threat may be so great that the work of reconciling is made more difficult than for women who have grown up with a more fatalistic sense that adversity is part of life and is to be accepted.

For other women, finding voice for their needs is a new and frightening project that had heretofore been hampered by limited self-knowledge and self-respect. Especially for women who have suffered abuse or neglect, recognizing and responding constructively to their own thoughts and feelings may be a new endeavor. Whether the abuse is the main issue that brings them to counseling or is uncovered along the path of other illness and loss, counselors will be faced with setting priorities as to which issues and behaviors to tackle first.

The primary tasks of normalizing will vary based on individual goals. For some women, working with uncertainty and bodily limitations is paramount, whereas for others, finding a way to express their feelings and desires to those around them is the largest task. Normalizing is a process rather than an outcome of adjusting to illness. It is what life is about after the initial reckoning and reconciling work is mostly done. Along the way emerges a life that includes but is not dominated by the demands of illness, that reflects a woman's unique gifts and abilities, and that engages support and integrates new information to make the best of ongoing challenges.

SUMMARY

After a serious blow to one's beliefs about life and the self, one can never fully return to the unconscious preillness state. Yet the outcome of reckoning and reconciling may be a life more fully lived than before, with greater awareness of both one's weaknesses and one's blessings. Women who have faced hurt and loss are more fully present to celebrate the possibilities that remain.

This chapter has presented a common pathway of illness recovery and some counseling implications. As we have noted, when any one of the four events of illness adjustment (suffering, reckoning, reconciling, normalizing) does not occur, distress may emerge later with serious health consequences. Counselors can assess women's progress along this path. They can support forward motion using skills of trust building, empathy, emotional awareness, self-esteem work, childhood review, self-inventorying and reappraisal, relationship work, cognitive-behavioral strategizing and repatterning, and role-playing for self-advocacy. As the uncertainties of an illness create new stressors and losses, an ongoing therapeutic relationship serves as an important buffer and workshop to maintain a woman's personalized sense of normalcy and selfhood in the face of threat and pain.

3

Cancer and Heart Disease

Responding to a Tragic Diagnosis

Many women are terrified at the thought of sudden serious illness. The two biggest killers of United States women, heart disease and cancer, strike hundreds of thousands of women each year. Cardiovascular disease causes one-half million deaths annually to women (Lemke, Pattison, Marshall, & Cowley, 1995, p. 251), about half of those due to coronary artery disease and the remainder due to stroke, congestive heart failure, or a combination. Yet cancer seems to be a greater fear for many women. Breast cancer is particularly frightening and is in fact the most common women's cancer, but lung cancer kills more women than does breast cancer, and heart disease kills more than twice as many women as all cancers combined (p. 191).

Our skewed conceptions about women's greatest health threats reflect the social and cultural meanings of these diseases, as well as the medical system's response to these illnesses in women. In this chapter, we will see how the personalized meanings of heart disease and cancer affect women's responses to these diagnoses. The life-changing nature of acute and potentially terminal illness is portrayed in women's reckoning with these diagnoses and becoming reconciled to their impacts on daily activities and the future.

HEART DISEASE: WOMEN'S GREATEST RISK

Women Don't Get Heart Attacks?

Heart disease affects a smaller proportion of women than men in the United States, yet women are more likely to die after heart attacks than are men (Lemke et al., 1995, p. 253). Women's rate of heart disease is low in their pre-menopausal years, but after age 50, their risk rises steeply to equal men's by the age of about 70. Women of color face a disproportionately higher risk of heart disease, as well as of other chronic diseases, such as diabetes and hypertension, that can lead to heart problems. This risk has been tied to poverty; lower education levels; high-salt, high-fat diet; and stress. White women with these risk factors also experience higher risk, yet discrimination in education, workplace, and health care settings and lack of health services in even well-to-do minority communities are added barriers to women of color. Lack of recognition and respect for culturally diverse value systems is a primary difficulty for black women, who are often treated as homogeneous, whether of African, Caribbean, South American, or other descent, and whether immigrant or native born (McBarnette, 1996, p. 45). Systematic oppression and disregard can lead to fatalism and lack of confidence in both health care and self-care.

Women's numerous and unending role responsibilities also have been found to push them along a different path in recovering from heart disease. Women are less likely than men to take time off, be passive, or allow themselves to be taken care of during their convalescence at home. They are less likely than men to attend cardiac rehabilitation programs. As they are more likely to outlive their spouses, women may not have spouse caregivers or the financial means to procure help during recovery. They may have older husbands who require much care themselves (Rankin, 1992). Women may not feel justified in refusing to perform household tasks or in seeking help for discomforting symptoms from physician authority figures (Hawthorne, 1993). For all these reasons, it is important to understand women's experiences of heart disease and their ways of coping with it, both to increase public attention to women's heart disease risk and to improve health professionals' response.

Surviving the Shock

Struggling with Symptoms for the Sake of Others

Many women disregarded their early heart attack symptoms. They didn't want to worry their loved ones, and they were uncomfortable relinquishing control of their bodies or their responsibilities to others. In interviews with a diverse group of women, Dempsey, Dracup, and Moser (1995) found that maintaining control was the women's chief objective in the period between noticing symptoms and coming in for treatment. Based on their lack of knowledge of women's symptoms and risk of cardiac disease and their personal experiences of previous illnesses, women tried to manage their own symptoms and continue their accustomed roles until the severity of their distress and the lack of effect of their self-care made it impossible to continue. An 82-year-old woman told them,

I didn't really think anything about it because I have arthritis so bad, a lot of times I do have pain. I thought, it's a trivial thing. (p. 449)

Even when symptoms seemed serious, women considered their commitments to others and concern for others' burdens. One remarked, "I didn't think it was anything serious. . . If I thought [my daughter] was out someplace then I wouldn't want to interrupt her day" (p. 450-451).

Hawthorne (1993) interviewed women recovering from coronary artery bypass surgery. They had interpreted their symptoms as not serious and not heart related. Some reported that their physicians made the same judgments. A black woman had sought help from her physician for her angina for 2 years:

I would just have, you know, sharp pains. . . through this left breast, and down into my arm. . . And he thought it was coming from a gas pocket that had developed in my gallbladder . . . I changed doctors and went to Dr. J. . . . And when she examined me, she told me that this was no gas bubble, this was my heart. (p. 231)

Cochrane (1992) also found that women were hampered in their early hours of symptoms by their own and others' lack of awareness of heart attack symptoms other than chest pain:

It was terrible, and it was all in my back . . . It didn't go down my left arm. That would have alerted me, I think, but it didn't go down like that. (p. 85)

Only about half of women with heart attacks have chest pain or discomfort (Rankin, 1992). The range of women's symptoms can include nausea and vomiting, jaw pain, arm pain, back pain, diarrhea, and general weakness or dizziness. With such an array of symptoms, women logically used remedies that seemed to address the symptom based on their experience, rather than concluding they were having heart attacks:

I thought it was muscular . . . I'd stop [sweeping the driveway] after about 15 or 20 minutes, and go in the house, and sit down, and watch the boob tube or something, and put the heating pad on my back. And it seemed to help. (Cochrane, 1992, p. 86)

When their symptoms did not respond to usual self-care measures or resembled what they knew about heart attacks, women sought help. Their first action, however, was most often not to contact a health professional but to check out their perceptions with a "lay consultant" (Dempsey et al., 1995). This could be a spouse, adult child, coworker, or friend. The consultants generally responded with immediate concern and action. Unfortunately, however, some did not. One woman was at work and was thought to be malingering to get out of working, and another's husband initially refused to respond to his wife's requests for help. Treatment was delayed, which increases the amount of heart damage and the risk of death (Dempsey et al., 1995).

Giving In to the Emergency

When symptoms persisted and self-care efforts failed to help, or when symptoms were severe or unfamiliar, women came to realize that they could not maintain control of them on their own and that outside help was needed. Some women felt great relief at no longer having to figure out what was wrong and what to do:

> I said, I don't feel good, and nothing else was said. He just took over. I felt better, because then he was in control. When I told my kids they called the paramedics. I knew they would know what to do to take care of it. (Dempsey et al., 1995, p. 452)

Once in the hands of medical professionals, many women found they were subjected to pain, indignity, and powerlessness, yet most endured this willingly for the sake of survival. In the hospital, they felt objectified; their bodies were handled as if they were mechanistic plumbing systems. They were confined and constrained, sometimes without understanding why. In interviews with women who had undergone cardiac surgery, King and Jensen (1994) found that in the hospital, women were focused on surviving the assaults to their accustomed roles and self-concepts:

> It was just all these horrible and humiliating things that were happening to me and I certainly didn't like it. You know . . . you do lose control. (p. 102)

Some patients used a strategy of distancing themselves from the seriousness of what had befallen them. In interviews with men and women after myocardial infarctions, Johnson and Morse (1990) reported that patients sought to demonstrate to themselves and others that they were not seriously ill by getting out of bed, concealing their pain, and joking. These were efforts to defend their normalcy in the face of increasing fear that they might die or their lives would be changed. They said that "everything seemed to be in a fog." (p. 129). The sedating and hallucinatory effects of medications increased women's difficulty in making sense of what was happening and grasping the impact of the heart attack on their future lives (King & Jensen, 1994).

Reckoning: Making Sense of the Breakdown

To accept the reality of their heart attacks and know what to do to prevent reoccurrence, women sought explanations for why they had happened. They became more aware of possible causes, although that did not always translate into changed behavior. Reast (1993) interviewed women in west Texas:

> I thought I was real healthy . . . I exercised. I walked an hour on my treadmill in here and we did watch our diet pretty well . . . I went to the doctor and the only thing I had was really a little high cholesterol. (p. 90)

When no clear explanation was found, stress often was considered a possible cause:

> None of my sisters have had heart attacks and I have [had] six. I guess I'm the only one. I don't think it's diet. I don't know what I did or didn't do. I was under stress at the time. I've been under stress before. (p. 91)

Women had a more difficult time than men in making sense of their heart attacks. They linked most risk factors to job-related stress.

A Wake-Up Call

Women in a support group for survivors of cardiac events questioned their personal values and beliefs about themselves and their world (Fleury et al., 1995). They felt vulnerable and confused:

> I feel like I am falling without a net. My old beliefs don't work anymore, but right now, I have nothing to replace them with. (p. 478)

Women who judged their heart attacks as life-changing events began to view time with new appreciation and think about shifting their priorities. They reviewed their habits and behaviors and considered what they would have to give up to reduce heart attack risk. They weighed the loss of pleasures such as eating rich food and smoking against the value of continued survival (Cochrane, 1992). Uncertainty about the cause of their illness, the vulnerability of their healing hearts, and the actual effectiveness of changing risky behaviors made the judgments more difficult.

In contrast with this call to action described by some women, others in different social and cultural contexts minimized the significance of their heart attacks. Hawthorne (1993), who studied men's responses to heart disease before interviewing women, found that women reacted much less strongly to the experience. This may have been due to the women's older age; they may have completed more of life's goals than had the men. They also were familiar with illness and caregiving and had helped others deal with death and loss. The lesser reaction also may have been due to their lack of comparable models in their social worlds. They had heard of hard-driving businessmen who needed to change their lifestyles after heart attacks, but they did not see themselves as having stressful work roles. Hawthorne's sample was drawn from the southern United States. She described the women as passive and deferent in their communication with health professionals and as having an "otherness" orientation that often led them to focus on others' needs rather than their own. In this cultural context, women viewed themselves as relatively powerless over their destinies.

Bodily Losses

The scars of heart surgery were extremely distressing to many women (Hawthorne, 1993). They experienced intense and prolonged pain from the incisions in their chests, made worse by the pressure of wearing a snug bra. Yet the pull of heavy breasts was even more painful. Women reported being unable to lift both arms at the same time, which meant they couldn't wash or comb their hair or fasten their bras behind them without acute discomfort. None had been warned of these obstacles by health professionals.

The disfigurement of the long, purple scars on chest and leg after bypass surgery led some women to feel devalued and unattractive. Again, this was more distressing for younger than for older women (King & Jensen, 1994).

I have a hangup about this scar on my chest. I have a horrible scar . . . It was a bad turn-off for L. I noticed that right off. I tried to get him to discuss it but he wouldn't. (p. 238)

Women were faced with taking stock of the damage once home from the hospital. Not only was the body scarred and painful; it was greatly weakened. Fatigue was a constant indicator of the heart's weakness, and it could be frightening to women who wondered whether their hearts would ever heal and whether they would be able to meet even the most basic responsibilities to their families, let alone rejoin activities they had pursued for pleasure.

The meaning of symptoms such as chest pain was difficult to assess:

Well, you always wonder. I mean, you're having the same pains. Is it heart-related? Is there something that they didn't [catch]? Did the angioplasty collapse? (Cochrane, 1992, p. 108)

In their recovery, women had to test their endurance and evaluate their symptoms in order to set up guidelines for themselves. As they sifted through information from doctors, family and friends, mass media, and other sources, they gradually developed personal understandings of what they could and could not do within their accustomed spheres of action.

Roles and Connections

Relationships were altered from the moment women relinquished control over their care and entered the health care system. Suddenly, others were doing for them, and they were powerless to give back. When they were at home and beginning to reconnect with loved ones and friends, some were met with a lack of emotional support or with surprise and distancing:

> My family treats me like a china doll. It's like they're afraid of me or something. They don't realize that I need them, and I won't break. (Fleury et al., 1995, p. 479)

On the other hand, many women found they were expected to resume their usual household duties and caregiving even beyond their immediate family. Some wanted to do so and expected it of themselves. When their physical fatigue and pain or the restrictions placed on them by health professionals prevented them from filling the perceived needs of others or from having their own newly understood needs met, they had to reassess the equity of exchange in family and friendships. Women wondered how to move from the primary caregiver role to a new role as a sometimes dependent partner (Fleury et al., 1995).

Reconciling: Remapping a Vulnerable Life

Caring for My Body and Caring for Myself

Based on their beliefs about the possibility of recovering a valued life, their understanding of what was necessary to reduce their risk of further heart disease, and their degree of commitment to advocating for themselves and their health, women began to seek ways to care for their vulnerable bodies and hearts. They made changes in their basic daily patterns of food and activity, to the degree they were able without intolerable disruption of family life.

In trying to follow instructions to cook with less fat, eat less meat, and consume more fruits, vegetables, and grains, women were faced with choices of adjusting the meals of those they cooked for, cooking more than one type of meal at once, giving up their program of change, or reneging on family meal preparation responsibilities. Some women who saw a pressing need to change their eating habits were able to do so by establishing their own health as a priority within the family and engaging other in part or all of the changes. Others who doubted the influence of diet on their health--or who were afraid or unwilling to challenge the patterns established in their families--had a harder time changing their food intake. Quitting smoking was another prescription that was difficult to follow in some family contexts. Women whose partners smoked were very doubtful that they would be able to quit until their partners did (Cochrane, 1992, p. 113).

Racial and cultural context affected women's understanding of and ability to comply with dietary recommendations. In social worlds where fried foods or baked desserts were expected at most meals, families were often reluctant to give these up, and women were often unwilling to ask them to. Likewise, their social contexts affected women's ability to consider seriously the recommendations of doctors. If women in their families had cooked and eaten rich foods for years and none other than themselves had become ill, women were less likely to believe in the importance of dietary changes.

Activity also was gauged by family needs and personal estimates rather than strictly by medical guidelines (Johnson & Morse, 1990). In early recovery, women used their fatigue (rather than professional advice) to decide what was safe and feasible physical activity (Fleury et al., 1995; Hawthorne, 1993). Progress was measured by which of their usual household tasks they were up to performing, although they did not always consider housework as "work" that should be paced. The cultural expectation of women to maintain the home environment was acutely felt. Some women felt unsupported in their need to rest and cut down on home maintenance, and others felt unduly restricted by physicians and family (Johnson & Morse, 1990). Some women felt so uncomfortable being idle that they sneaked around in order to feel that they were contributing to the household:

> Last week when nobody was here, I did a load of laundry by myself. "Oh-oh . . . my son is looking around the corner." . . . There was a bunch of stuff in the clothes hamper . . . I just want to help a little bit. (Cochrane, 1992, p. 112)

Yet in later recovery, when they were advised by health professionals to increase exercise beyond their accustomed level to strengthen their hearts, some had no personal experience of vigorous exercise--of fitting it into their lives or judging how much fatigue was safe. Their compliance with this instruction depended a great deal on support of family members and their own understandings of and beliefs in the importance of exercise. It was viewed as a prescription at first, rather than recreation:

> [My husband] keeps track of every walk we take, how much. He keeps track of the pills that I take. . . . And then he walks with me every day. (Cochrane, 1992, p. 112)

In adjusting their activities for their healing hearts, women's personal guidelines evolved out of compromises between what they were told and what they felt they could realistically achieve while maintaining important aspects of their relationships and commitments.

Am I Different?

Looking back at their brush with death, women worked to integrate this new information about themselves with the person they had been and what they were capable of. The younger the woman, the greater the impact. The idea of being vulnerable, of having a weak heart, was harder to adjust to for women who had seen themselves as having many years to live, and as healthy and taking good care of themselves. It was easier for those who had accepted other illnesses and the unpredictability of their life spans. Life became more valuable and meaningful for many. It became more discouraging for a few who were unable to reconcile this new information with the person they had been and expected to be.

New priorities emerged. "It's like cutting to the center of things, you realize what is important now. Unimportant things fall away" (Fleury et al., 1995, p. 479). New strength was found when women stood up to prior expectations of themselves and others, advocating for their new goals. Some claimed time for themselves to exercise or rest and limited their involvement in social engagements or family disputes that were draining and unrewarding. Each priority-setting achievement was seen as evidence of new personal power. Recovery from a heart attack was simultaneously facing vulnerability and identifying new strengths. As a result, a woman redefined her self-worth based on who she was and what she could accomplish for herself, and less on physical tasks she could do for others:

> You think about what's your good point. You know what my good point is, I'm the best listener in the world. . . . When I was up to see my friend . . . we had to go over [to see a woman with multiple sclerosis] for tea. And mind you, I've only met this woman once before, so we went over. And you know, you felt so good when you left, because I knew I had sat and listened to her. . . . She just gets so lonesome. (Cochrane, 1992, p. 155)

Balancing Relationships

After a cardiac event, women who reset their priorities often needed to look for new ways to cooperate with others rather than returning to the role of caretaker. They asked for help, or paid for it, although often with ambivalence at this new delegation of their responsibilities:

You're so used to doing everything yourself. I've always been independent. I don't know, it can't be all bad having somebody come in and clean house for you. (Cochrane, 1992, p. 111)

They also balanced their emotional work and caregiving of others. Many pulled back from over-investment in draining relationships and restructured their obligations when unable to meet them given their newfound priorities. For older couples, dual illnesses required major readjustments in caregiving, especially for women whose self-definition had been tied up in meeting physical and emotional needs of others.

Some women felt unable to advocate for their own needs in their households or families or unwilling to disrupt what felt like a tenuous relationship, or they lived alone and unsupported without financial means to hire help. This was a different kind of reconciling: making peace with the fact that although they faced a health risk, other pressures were stronger.

Over time, normalizing one's life after heart attack meant making the new changes part of a personalized, stable, and manageable lifestyle. Women who took on and persisted in major changes found ongoing reward in their successful adjustment to the challenge of maintaining a new diet, exercise, and ways of relating. Some were able to celebrate their newly expanded coping abilities. They were more comfortable with their scars and limitations and found that their new humility was balanced with a new pride in themselves and appreciation of life. Having learned the value of support and assistance in their own daily obligations, some reached out to others to give support and offered help when they were able (Cochrane, 1992; Fleury et al., 1995). But for women who did not accept the importance or efficacy of personal lifestyle changes or did not view their heart conditions as serious, normalizing meant going on with life as they had before, despite the threat and disruption of illness.

Adjusting to Heart Disease: Counselors' Roles

The risk of not reckoning with or reconciling to the demands of heart disease is relapse or death. A few women who were interviewed had not fully reckoned with the losses implied in their heart attacks (Cochrane, 1992; Johnson & Morse, 1990) because they were not given or were unable to understand the facts of their situation. Or they had absorbed the significance of their risk but were too threatened by its meaning or lacked the personal resources to reconcile it with their lives.

These are the women most in need of counseling work and least likely to seek help. Like addicts who don't acknowledge that their drug use is a problem, some women may be unable to see the importance of making major changes after a heart attack. These women may come to counselors for other reasons, such as anxiety or difficulty dealing with family stress. They need concrete yet compassionate evidence of their risk and help putting family demands into perspective. Work on strengthening self-esteem and hope and identifying and bolstering supports may enable some of these women eventually to take on the challenge of learning about and adjusting to their heart disease. Cognitive work, role-playing, or family counseling may help women advocate for themselves effectively within tense family environments. Social service referrals may be needed to engage household help or health services to relieve women of caregiving and housework burdens. Emotional support and empathy can strengthen women's faith in their own abilities to change their priorities and protect their futures.

CANCER: THE GREATEST FEAR

Cancer is the second most common cause of death in women. The 5-year survival rates for all cancers averages 53% (Meyerowitz & Hart, 1995). Breast cancer is the most common type of cancer diagnosed in women, followed by lung and colon cancer, but lung and colon cancer kill more of their victims. Preventive and early detection measures have not reached poor communities and women of color, although they have become easily accessible to white women (McBarnette, 1996). For this reason and perhaps because of lesser use of health services due to cultural differences in meanings of illness, women of color and poor women have a greater risk of being diagnosed at an advanced stage of cancer (Mathews, Lannin, & Mitchell, 1994) and of dying of the disease.

Most cancers are much more common in women after menopause. Yet cancer is feared by many young women, perhaps because when it does occur in relatively young women still active in employment and raising families, it intrudes so visibly and tragically. Some cancers, such as breast, uterine, and cervical cancer, are quite curable if diagnosed early, whereas others such as pancreatic, ovarian, and lung cancer have poor prognoses. However, regardless of the site of cancer, the word carries frightening emotional meanings. Women familiar with the medical aspects of cancer treatment associate it with disfiguring surgery, painful, debilitating chemotherapy and radiation treatments, and ultimately, with slow, painful death.

Reckoning with Cancer: Uncertain Self in a Changed World

My Body Against Me: The Meaning of Cancer

In contrast to heart disease, which often came upon women unaware and demanded attention as a sudden acute illness event, women interviewed by researchers reported that cancer often had a more insidious onset. It often included a tense, protracted diagnostic period, followed by surgery, chemotherapy, radiation, or all three. For many women, cancer meant a threat of death. Regardless of the cure rates or likelihood of long-term control of the disease, the diagnosis represented a capricious and terrifying turning of the body against itself and against all that had been hoped for in the future.

As women began to reckon with the diagnosis of cancer, their bodies became a source of uncertainty and threat. In interviews with women who had survived invasive cervical cancer (Leonard, 1990), each remembered with clarity the moment of receiving their cancer diagnosis, and the immediate connotation of early death:

> When they told me that, I said that must mean I'm going to die because everybody who had cancer that I ever heard of was going to die. . . . I found out on a Thursday at three o'clock. (p. 68)

Cultural context shaped the meaning of being told one had cancer. The predominant medical metaphor of cancer is that the disease is a wily enemy to be fought against using an arsenal of high-tech weapons. By contrast, southern African American women with advanced breast cancer (Mathews et al., 1994) made sense of the problem using indigenous definitions of illness, such as an imbalance in the blood or entrapment of dirty blood in the system. Early symptoms were linked to changes in the blood:

> That knot I had came and went. If you have dirty blood, the impurities have to go somewhere. And once I passed the change, that blood just stayed in me all the time. . . . When I fell down that day in the garden, they all came up to that bruise and they made a lump. (p. 793)

The knot or root of bad blood could take on a life and growth of its own over time. If cure was to be found, it would come from the power of the Lord:

> When you have cancer, then there's nothing for it but to turn it over to God. If you have enough faith, He will heal it and you don't need no operation. Because there is nothing a doctor can do for you--Only God has the power. (p. 795)

Given the lack of human role in the cure, the logical response was to leave the lump alone to avoid stirring it up. Only when the black women were persuaded to take part in conventional treatment did their stories begin to combine their earlier understandings with the medical metaphors of being a partner in the fight against disease.

Enduring New Treatment With Old Ways of Coping

As cancer treatment began, women fell back on their accustomed outlooks and coping strategies to get through it. A group of diverse women who were undergoing chemotherapy for breast cancer (Berman, 1993) had three ways of focusing on illness. Many women were able to maintain an integrated focus, balancing the demands of cancer treatment with the rest of life. These women were resilient, balanced, and did not find chemotherapy a huge disruption. Some women had a centralized focus: Cancer was the main content of their lives at that point. They were having severe side effects and felt less hopeful than the others about survival. The third way of focusing was segmented: Women whose lives were already unstable and demanding found that they were overwhelmed by cancer on top of other demands and inadequate resources, and they felt the need to address all of their concerns at once. They were exhausted by the pileup of demands, although chemotherapy side effects were not a central focus of their concern. These three outlooks on cancer were unrelated to the woman's seriousness of disease or to cultural or socioeconomic differences.

Similarly, in women with advanced breast or ovarian cancer undergoing chemotherapy without expectation of cure, Payne (1990) found that some women took a "think positive" stance and sought to use their strength to fight for their lives, refusing to stop planning for the future even when they knew their condition was terminal. Others took an accepting stance, tolerating the recurrence of their cancer and seeking to simply make the best of it for the time they had left. A third group reacted with behavior of extreme fearfulness, displaying tense, rigid postures, wanting to live at all costs, yet abdicating all decision making. The fourth group felt hopeless, felt that cancer had taken over, and became dependent on others to manage their treatment, not wanting to know about the details yet unable to focus on anything but their disease.

In a third example of differing outlooks, Kesselring (1990) interviewed women undergoing chemotherapy for initial or recurrent breast cancer. Some of these women viewed their lives as merely "on hold" during cancer treatment, fully expecting to resume most aspects afterward. They were mainly wives of successful professionals. They grieved most acutely their loss of certainty and control. Some younger women took a more intellectual, probabilistic view of their situations and actively participated in treatment, as partners with medical professionals. They continued their work responsibilities simultaneously with managing chemotherapy. Kesselring also identified two women, one Asian and the other white, with less education and income than the others in her sample but with close family networks, who saw cancer as a disease that would take its course regardless of action on their part. These women experienced their selves and bodies as in unity and viewed their roles in life as family members rather than as independent actors. They did not project into the future or intellectualize about odds of survival or their personal contributions to the course of disease.

In a fourth study, Kagan (1994) interviewed older cancer sufferers, women and men with an average age of 74. In general, these older individuals did not see cancer as a major life-threatening emergency, given the long and complex and already much-completed history of their lives. The women had three different patterns of integrating cancer into their lives. Some were "confident that I'll beat it," not letting life be overtaken by cancer; others "don't think about it," viewing other illnesses and issues as more pressing than cancer; and still others viewed cancer as "another piece of the puzzle," a new but not surprising burden in a long accumulation of debilitating illnesses. In each of these studies, during cancer treatment women judged its degree of life change and burden in the context of their already constructed worldviews. Only after treatment did the reckoning and reconciling process begin in earnest.

Living in a Different Body

Cancer treatment, including chemotherapy and radiation, made the body completely undependable for periods of time as women endured the extreme fatigue, nausea, insomnia, and pain of treatment. Some women treated for cervical cancer struggled with loss of bowel and bladder control that persisted long after the treatment (Leonard, 1990). It became impossible to rely on their bodies to do what had previously been effortless and spontaneous: walk to the bathroom, cook dinner, hold a conversation with friends. They experienced the world differently. Distances seemed longer, and time seemed either longer or shorter, more precious or more boring. Some wondered, Is this the beginning of the end? Their bodies were simultaneously disturbingly unreliable parts of themselves and separate entities from their thoughts and feelings. A woman offered up her body into the hands of medical professionals for invasive treatment, deterrence of cancer and its symptoms with drugs, and ongoing analysis of its status with powerful tests (Kesselring, 1990).

> [In the beginning] you're very threatened: the "you" is threatened, the essence of you. Everything that you know about you is changing. It's being swept out from under you, and you don't know what's going to happen. (Leonard, 1990, p. 69)

The loss of the taken-for-granted body was a central aspect of the cancer experience (Kesselring, 1990). For many women, the body lost its familiar contours and capacities as a result of cancer and its treatment. They were faced with adjusting to missing breasts and loss of hair:

> People at work have kind of clichés of, well: "you know it's just a useless gland," "it's not who you are." And . . . I know it's not who I am but still I feel like I'm going to be mutilated, so I don't like it. (Kesselring, 1990, p.

162)

> It's bad enough losing your breast, which I can hide. But I sure can't hide my head. (Berman, 1993, p. 49)

Women who had hysterectomies for cervical cancer also grieved, although their loss was less visible:

> You've had a loss, so you have to cope with that. . . . a loss of time, maybe six months or a year . . . when you couldn't be the way you used to be. And then in my case I had a loss of my body part which physically is very demanding but also emotionally. (Leonard, 1990, p. 74)

Impact on Relationships

The changed body, the demands of treatment, and the uncertainty of survival also affected women's relationships, revealing to them ways they used support and ways they didn't want to use help.

> We just got closer. Maybe he grew up more, but it just seemed to happen at the time that I got cancer. . . . He just stayed home with me. . . . We expressed our feelings to each other which we never did so much before. . . . Something clicked in him like, "Gee, maybe I'm going to lose her." (Leonard, 1990, p. 73)

Some women who were single or widowed felt the absence of intimate support:

> When you're single . . . there tends not to be anyone you can talk to in a really specific way. . . . Mostly when they're married women, their husbands are very involved in the decisions. (Leonard, 1990, p. 70)

> I would love to have come home and kind of cried to somebody. And . . . it would only be a husband. (Kagan, 1994, p. 116)

Yet, women also experienced difficulties with others' desires to be intimate or helpful, and they had to deal with others' grief as well as their own uncertainty. The most painful worry to deal with was their children's future.

> [I] worried about what I can't do, preventing me from doing things--working and driving . . . because I am very self-reliant and self-sufficient. Being dependent on other people really bothers me. (Kesselring, 1990, p. 193)

> "Mummy are you going to die?" and stuff like that. I said, "No, I'm not going to die"--not knowing myself whether I was or not . . . and maybe it was even then that I made up my mind that I wasn't going to. (Leonard,

1990, p. 71)

Older women experienced much less impact from cancer diagnosis and treatment than did younger women. Kagan (1994) noted that in reckoning with cancer, they conducted an internal dialogue with the self, and most came to the conclusion that cancer was a relatively minor threat in the context of a life mostly lived (p. 81).

Rewriting the Future

The inner dialogue women conducted as they reckoned with cancer involved rewriting their personal biographies (Corbin & Strauss, 1988; Wiener & Dodd, 1993). Their bodies were inextricable from their views of their past, present, and future; their understandings and assumptions of what they had been and done and would be and do in the future were radically changed by cancer. The past became newly appreciated or regretted, depending on whether it had been lived fruitfully and rewardingly or dissipated in less valued ways. The present was altered due to the impact of physical illness on daily life and interaction.

The future was most grievously changed and was characterized by uncertainty. Accepting this uncertainty was probably the most difficult aspect of cancer for many women. The younger the woman, the greater the impact on her future. This processing often occurred during periods of great physical distress and debility, yet the intermissions between cycles of chemotherapy or radiation brought back feelings of health and well-being, which only increased the women's uncertainty about what was ahead in the longer term.

Reconciling to a New Body and Biography

Coping with Symptoms and Body Changes

Women revealed their different coping styles in their approaches to practical matters of managing the physical effects of cancer and the internal work of dealing with its impact. Some experienced minimal disruption because their symptoms were relatively mild, or they were determined not to let cancer and its treatment interfere with their other life priorities. Other women were devastated by side effects of chemotherapy or radiation or interpreted their bodily changes as extreme threats to their selfhood and ability to go on living. Based on these widely varying assessments, women moved forward to integrate these changes into self and relationships.

Women who were accustomed to planning, as a strategy for controlling intrusions into their lives, found themselves planning for the impact of chemotherapy:

> I just think about the chemotherapy, and how best to deal with it. Because it is a time-consuming, a thought-consuming process. Because, it requires so many days from when you feel really great to when you feel really great again. And then you know you just have that certain time before you know it starts all over again. So, what can you accomplish in that time, how many things can I do. So, it's something you have to work around. (Berman, 1993, p. 51)

When unable to control symptoms, women accustomed to being able to continue their usual lives by force of determination felt frightened and dismayed:

> I just can't believe this, that I just cannot make myself feel better. It was one of the most frustrating things in the world because throughout the ten, twelve years [of cancer] I've just been able to grit myself into doing better and [this time] I really couldn't. I lost 18 pounds in 10 days. I had no energy at all. (Kesselring, 1990, p. 128)

Thresholds for discomfort and disability varied, depending on the illness severity and treatment plan but also on women's backgrounds and cultures. For some, the physical assaults of cancer treatment were overwhelming and for others, a minor annoyance. Some women experienced pain from mouth sores, stomach upset, or skin sores during chemotherapy or radiation, but in early cancer, pain was usually temporary. Women with recurrent and metastatic cancer endured greater and more continuous pain and with it the bodily message that the disease was spreading. They juggled the relief brought by medication with the accompanying loss of alertness, seeking to find the point of balance between freedom from pain and loss of ability to observe and participate in their lives.

Music, relaxation, distraction, prayer, staying in bed, and other ways of coping with pain, nausea, and fatigue were ways to minimize the disruptions of their illness.

> I prepared myself to be sick. And I had the Compazine [anti-nausea medication] out and I had everything by my bed that, if I was going to throw up, and throw up in a hurry, that I would be in bed and I would be able to decide. (p. 118)

> But anyway, we always had music. So I went in and turned the TV on or the radio on, and I enjoyed it so much. . . . And, of course, prayer. I'm not overly religious. but, especially when I go to bed at night and I try to get to sleep, I try to pray. And that helps too. (Kagan, 1994, p. 117)

In public, disfigurement was dealt with by practical means, including breast prostheses, wigs, and scarves. Yet these efforts felt counterproductive to some women who sought to accept their changed bodies and have others do the same. A woman concealed or revealed her changes depending on her desired self-image and the response she expected from others. Minimizing changes in appearance to avoid stigma and pity was a priority for some, whereas others wanted to demonstrate that they were at peace with or even proud of their changed appearance.

Adjusting Relationships

Relationships with loved ones required profound changes on all levels. Sexual intimacy was made difficult by concern about their changed body, surgical incisions, and fatigue. There could be vaginal soreness after treatment for cervical cancer:

> For a while I felt irritated every time my husband tried to touch me . . . it would be all I could do to hold back from just telling him to get away from me. But I've kind of learned to cope with it. (Leonard, 1990, p. 73)

In the more mundane aspects of shared responsibilities and pleasures, many women were periodically unable to do household chores during the cycles of chemotherapy, meaning that some spouses took on these tasks for the first time in addition to their burdens of maintaining financial stability and worrying about their wives. Communication became critical as couples repatterned intimate relationships. When it was strained or conflicted, women felt alone and unsupported, and unsure of how to proceed.

With the onset of the demands of cancer treatment, some women reconsidered their more peripheral acquaintanceships and let go some that were more burdensome than helpful. With ongoing friends, they discussed the illness most at its onset and then only brought it up when something new was happening. Friends then reciprocally would follow up on the new developments, which helped to diffuse the shared worry (Kagan, 1994).

Managing Uncertainty

Much of the work of reconciling with cancer was finding ways to deal with fear, doubt, and lack of knowledge about the success of treatment and what the future would bring. Women described a variety of cognitive strategies for keeping uncertainty at bay (Hinds & Martin, 1988; Kagan, 1994; Payne, 1990; Wiener & Dodd, 1993). These efforts included reducing awareness through distraction by deliberately thinking of something else or getting involved in activities; pacing themselves to save energy for valued activities and avoid breakdown; setting goals such as looking forward to a wedding or simply the end of treatment; minimization or seeking reinforcing comparisons in order to see oneself as better off than other sufferers; prayer and faith practices (Mathews et al., 1994); and humor, even in the face of clearly terminal illness, which lightened mood and made fun of the seriousness with which their situation was often regarded. "The times I feel the best are the times when I'm serene in spite of whatever is going on" (Kesselring, 1990, p. 267).

Other strategies included keeping up appearances, both physical and emotional, concealing fear, sadness, and other negative emotions until there was a safe place to let down one's guard and be vulnerable; and wishful thinking, indulging oneself in thoughts of cure and longevity even when this was unlikely, simply for the emotional comfort it brought. Another type of strategy against uncertainty was taking charge, becoming expert in the disease, holding the reins in treatment decisions, directing the running of the household and work responsibilities even from one's bed, and seeking to master one's body through willpower, while also protecting it from undue assaults by medical professionals. Women's lifelong patterns of coping determined which of these strategies were most accessible and useful.

An important strategy was seeking and using support. For some women, this was their first thought and their most important source of help. The sources of helpful support varied according to the women's outlooks. Those who saw their conditions as temporary sought help from intimates and friends and did not use support groups, whereas women experiencing recurrent cancer found these groups helpful and sometimes essential.

Strategies for Facing Death

The challenge of reconciling to death overwhelmed old coping patterns. The mind-over-matter cognitive strategies with which some women bolstered their senses of control and mastery broke down (Kesselring, 1990). At this point, reasoning lost its utility and importance, and women focused more on making peace with their failing bodies and less on controlling or fighting against them. Despair came with giving up the sense of self-determination, but for some, it was followed by peace and understanding when they were able to reframe their situation as part of a larger plan.

> In my whole life, I never learned how to be happy and then I got cancer, and because of the [spiritual] work we've been doing, I've been happy. It's ironic . . . I go through my periods of wondering if I'm dying . . . my periods of being very sad, depressed, angry, whatever--the whole spectrum of emotions . . . but generally speaking, I feel really happy. (Kesselring, 1990, p. 268)

Likewise, adolescents with cancer described achieving periods of cognitive comfort when they could see that life was larger than their disease.

All of a sudden I realize that I haven't been thinking about cancer. I've just been thinking about regular stuff. Then I feel so good because I know that there's more to me than being sick with cancer. That's when I get real hopeful. (Hinds & Martin, 1988, p. 339)

In these peaceful times, the teenagers were able to apply this hope to even very painful issues, such as how their parents would fare if they died or whether their own strength would hold out so that they could bear up under treatment and give hope to younger cancer patients. Likewise, mature women were able to find hope and peace when they looked beyond the present illness to see themselves in a larger scheme and envision how life would continue even without their influence or witness.

Normalizing Life with Cancer: Balancing Living and Dying

Living with cancer meant balancing the demands of illness and treatment, of everyday lives, and of revising one's internal biography. It meant maintaining the important aspects of living (Kagan, 1994) even as one dealt with the ongoing burdens of illness and worked to reconcile oneself to possible early death (Wiener & Dodd, 1993). Women accepted new thresholds of activity and participation in former roles--for some, temporary, and for others, more permanent.

Women who had completed treatment and were deemed cured described it as "reclaiming their bodies" (Leonard, 1990). They took over where health professionals had formerly acted, taking on the tasks of watching for symptoms and judging recovery and of making sense of what had befallen them and the implications for their future. Some spoke of wanting to tell their stories to help other women.

Younger women who completed chemotherapy for breast cancer (Berman, 1993) saw themselves as moving on to a life that was in many ways the same as the one they had before cancer but in some ways changed. They spoke of looking back at the treatment experience with relief that it had not been as bad as they had expected but with awareness that it was a wake-up call to reexamine their priorities. They also looked forward and realized they could not plan for the future with the degree of certainty they had formerly assumed. Cancer would be a constant shadow for the rest of their lives. Some women were grateful for their relatively easy course and wanted to support other women through similar experiences.

Young women who survived breast cancer and went on to have children also shifted their focus from the imprecise future to the here and now. They explained that they chose to take a medical risk and have children because it was their highest priority, after staying alive. Motherhood enabled them to regain a sense of normalcy, to reconnect with the cycle of life and other women who were mothers, and to invest in the future. Some undertook this project in spite of warnings from doctors that pregnancy could prompt a recurrence of cancer (Dow, 1994).

Even in terminal cancer, living for at least the near future remained as important as dying. In a study of married couples in which the wife's breast cancer had recurred, couples actively worked to keep cancer a background rather than a foreground issue (Lewis & Deal, 1995). While they watched for new symptoms and sought to interpret them and acknowledged periods of sadness and uncertainty, the couples focused on survival and even healing. They deliberately avoided dwelling on difficult topics of conversation, including plans for dying and after death.

Although this brought peace within the relationship, it took its toll on the individuals. Wives were more interested in talking about what would happen after their deaths than were their husbands. Some felt their husbands were unable to handle their wives' sadness and fear, and these women reserved these feelings for support group peers. Yet these coping strategies did not always relieve these relationships of strain. In 60% of these couples, one or both members were depressed or dissatisfied with their marriages (Lewis & Deal, 1995).

Counseling Women With Cancer

Unlike heart disease sufferers, cancer patients are more likely to seek or be offered help to cope with the psychological aspects of their disease, because we recognize cancer's life-threatening and body-image-changing nature. Women with cancer spend much more time in contact with treatment providers than do those who are recovering from heart attacks. When counseling can continue over a period of time, it has the potential to provide a context for deep review of a woman's life and for restructuring of her sense of herself, her roles, relationships, and the future, for greater peace of mind and sense of coherence.

In working with women with cancer, counselors will encounter a variety of ways of viewing the disease and its treatment, from the most mastery oriented to the most passive and accepting, the very optimistic or denying of threat, to the overwhelmed and despairing. The challenge will be to preserve each woman's sense of stability and continuity within her life context while opening up new avenues for self-understanding and growth. Gathering up-to-date information from doctors and nurses about the components and choices of treatment and their likely effects and success will bolster counselors' frames of reference and help them support women's own emotion-laden understandings.

Body Image Issues

With cancer's threats to the body and the self, counselors can expect women to struggle with losses of physical beauty, wholeness, symmetry, and reliability. Work such as imagery, body mapping, role playing, and desensitization may greatly enhance a woman's ability to reckon with and reunite with a changed physical self. Equally powerful can be meeting other women who are confident and vibrant despite losses of breasts or hair. Feelings of sadness and hopelessness can intensify women's grief over their changed bodies, and work on depression may be needed. Likewise, fatigue and nausea can feed into depression; insight into the cyclic patterns of uplift that can come after the devastating days of treatment may enable women to retain bits of hope for feeling better even in the depths of distressing symptoms.

Establishing a warm, accepting relationship is the basic platform on which more difficult work can occur. Women who feel inadequate and unlovable due to their altered bodies will need a safe, nurturing counseling environment. They must to come to terms with and reintegrate with their scars and disfigurement before they will be able to take on the more long-term threats of their illness. Counselors can persist in providing positive regard, identifying strengths and assets while acknowledging with candor the real changes women are facing.

Obligations to Loved Ones

Women with cancer struggle to accept their reduced abilities to contribute to household income and tasks, and to events and recreation in the workplace and among friends and family. Mealtimes, formerly the time of reconnecting and sharing pleasure, may become ordeals to be avoided, as nausea, fatigue, and mouth sores make eating something to be feared. Finding other ways to be part of family gatherings, exchanges, and communication is an important task. Counselors can elicit ideas about other ways families can operate and share time together while preserving what is most important about family rituals and traditions. Communication strategies may be critically important in conflicted or distant families when cancer further strains these links. Women may need help to devise other sources of support, such as friends, support groups, clergy, or counselors, if families are unable to provide the accepting companionship that is needed.

The threat of death is felt not only as a burden on a woman's own hopes and dreams but as a harm she is inflicting on those closest to herself. Women with cancer may need help coping with uncertainty about future family participation, be it earning a living to support children, being there for important milestones, or being able to guide and nurture young children or share old age with a spouse. Guilt, fear, regret, and sadness are especially poignant with respect to relationships. Ventilation and catharsis may be available only in the safe space of a counseling relationship. Cognitive restructuring may also be helpful when women are unwilling to share any of their illness experience for fear of hurting others. Enhancing reciprocity in relationships can be a positive outcome of illness-related work.

Lewis and Deal's 1995 study of couples in which the wife had recurrent breast cancer revealed that unwillingness to confront the reality of terminality was adaptive to a certain extent, in that it enabled these families to go on with their lives. The authors suggested that support may be better offered by eliciting reflections on illness experiences rather than introducing "reality testing" when clearly a woman is near death. At the same time, they noted that sad feelings clearly do not go away. Women and their families need to be encouraged to listen to and accept each other's fears and grief.

Existential Questions

Women who never before considered the meaning of life, their degree of self-determination, or the importance of longevity versus quality of life may bring these deep concerns to counseling sessions. Illness may call for restructuring of beliefs and faith or reconnection with a religious tradition. Spiritual practice may bring a kind of solace available nowhere else. Counselors may be able to guide women toward resources within existing religious traditions, to books and films in which other cancer patients discuss these concerns, or to development of new practices, such as meditation, contemplation, or new forms of prayer.

Connecting With Others Like Me

Last but very important is the counselors' role in connecting women with cancer to support groups and advocacy groups where they can give and receive support among others who understand their inner ordeal. Providing names and phone numbers, describing what happens in a support group and what women have gained from them, and framing their participation as a contribution to others if not a source of aid to themselves may help women take steps to explore this potential source of support. Participating in advocacy groups, such as those in which breast cancer survivors meet with recently diagnosed women, may enable a woman with cancer to make a meaningful contribution and be connected to others. She may establish new friendships. Both new and long-term cancer sufferers can benefit from proactive peer outreach and support.

CONCLUSIONS

Although different in their cultural meanings and clinical trajectories, heart disease and cancer are the most common killers of women in the United States. In each illness, women suffer with physical, emotional, and interpersonal threats until they are able to reckon with the impacts of the disease on their selves and social worlds and find ways to reconcile these losses with their persisting selves. Then life-threatening illness can recede to become just one part of a normal life. Counselors help women sustain faith in their own value and their ability to come to terms with uncertainty and disfigurement and use a repertoire of strategies to endure pain and suffering while focusing on what of importance remains.

Both cancer and heart disease may move from acute crisis phases into a chronic illness pattern, in which women live for years with physical limitations and uncertainty about the future. In the next chapter we explore other chronic illnesses and examine how women respond to health threats that persist over time.

4

Learning to Live With It

Integrating Self and Chronic Illness

Chronic illness is progressive, recurrent, and enduring (Gregg, Robertus, & Stone, 1989). Illnesses that come to stay, rather than being short-term visitors, require extensive restructuring of understandings of who we are, what our work and home lives will be like, how people will interact with us, how we will survive financially, and how we will manage daily life around the symptoms of illness and care for its demands. Common chronic illnesses include diabetes, arthritis, multiple sclerosis, kidney disease, high blood pressure, and HIV. Cancer and heart disease become chronic when the acute life threat is controlled but the adjustment to the disease is ongoing. There are also chronic disabilities due to injury or internal events, such as stroke, that leave their victims physically disabled.

The processes of dealing with chronic illness has been described by researchers such as Strauss (e.g., Corbin & Strauss, 1988) and Charmaz (e.g., 1991), and readers particularly interested in chronic illness are encouraged to consult their work. Particular attention will be given here to illnesses common to women and women's statements about their experiences. We will focus on two illnesses for which a fair amount of information is available about women's experience: diabetes and multiple sclerosis. We also will hear from women with fibromyalgia, a still poorly understood condition of muscle pain and overwhelming fatigue.

Diabetes, the inability to produce enough insulin to keep blood sugar in a normal range, affects approximately 11 million Americans; 90% have Type II diabetes, which usually begins in middle age, and about 10% have Type I, which often begins in childhood or adolescence. The disease is slightly more common in men than in women, yet women are more likely to experience long-term complications of eye damage, heart disease, and high blood pressure (Barrett-

Connor & Wingard, 1984). Diabetes is the third most common cause of death in the United States, and persons with Type I diabetes may not live more than two-thirds their expected lifespan. About 75% of those with Type I diabetes die of heart or kidney failure due to their diabetes. The complications can be staved off somewhat by scrupulous attention to maintaining blood sugar within a narrow range, which requires frequent self-testing, insulin injections, and dietary and exercise control. Some persons with Type II diabetes can control blood sugar by diet and oral medications without insulin injections (Gregg et al., 1989).

Multiple sclerosis (MS) affects approximately 350,000 persons in the United States (Anderson et al., 1992), 65% of whom are women and are white. MS is a disease of the nervous system, in which the myelin coating of the central nervous system becomes inflamed and degenerates, interfering with signals from the brain to the rest of the body. It strikes young adults in cold climates most commonly and can produce mild or totally disabling symptoms that come and go unpredictably but can be triggered by stressful events. These symptoms can include vision loss, loss of coordination and balance, weakness and dizziness, pain and numbness, loss of bladder control, and extreme fatigue. There is no known cure, and treatment is focused on reducing the harm and discomfort of the symptoms (Gregg et al., 1989).

A woman with a chronic illness soon discovers that health care systems are generally designed for acute care, often leaving chronically ill patients to advocate for themselves in the maze of agencies and regulations (Thorne, 1993). Likewise, governmental protections have only recently been extended to chronically disabled persons, and then only after extensive activism by the disabled themselves. The Americans With Disabilities Act, passed in 1990, mandates that the private sector make reasonable accommodation for the physically and mentally disabled in access to employment, products, and services (Lubkin, 1995).

Social and cultural accommodation still falls short of integrating the chronically ill into many arenas of American life. It can be difficult to accommodate the chronically ill in a work environment where consistent performance and emotional stability are expected. We have conflicting expectations for the behavior of the ill person. On one hand, we expect her to accept her limitations, comply with medical restrictions and instructions, and appreciate the help of others. On the other hand, we expect her to work extremely hard to overcome her limitations and change habits that may be unhealthy or contributing to the disease. When a man is ill, we tend to think of his personal loss of career and future, but when a woman is ill, we think first of others' loss--her children and family--and only later may consider what it means to her to be unable to work. We expect emotion focused coping from women and stoic cognitive problem solving from men. Yet, all these issues and responses affect both men and women.

The reckoning and reconciling process as it works in chronic illness requires coming to terms with the betrayal of the body and the failure of American culture and health systems to make illness an acceptable part of life; facing impairment and the changes it brings into identity, work, and relationships in daily life; and dealing with recurring grief and frustration in the up-and-down process of rebuilding a new version of normal life.

RECKONING: LEARNING THE SHAPE OF CHRONIC ILLNESS

Diagnosis as Life-Changing Event

Although symptoms can be painful, embarrassing, and frightening, what they mean can be even more distressing. Only with a culturally coherent understanding of what is causing the problem and what is expected for the future can women reckon with what is lost. With a diagnosis comes information and often relief of uncertainty. Until a diagnosis is identified, women with unexplained symptoms are alone and in limbo. Some illnesses are not readily diagnosed, which can mean months or years coping with unexplained symptoms and the fear of what they might mean. Women with fibromyalgia and multiple sclerosis often described this course. Diabetes, on the other hand, was easily identified for most women.

Diabetes can have a sudden onset with excessive thirst, frequent urination, and hunger, or even coma, or it can have a gradual start and be identified at a routine screening. Usually, diabetes that begins in childhood or young adulthood (Type 1) involves sudden loss of the ability to produce insulin with a fairly dramatic onset of symptoms, whereas diabetes that begins in later adulthood (Type 2) involves increased insulin needs, often due to obesity, and resistance of the body to insulin, causing high blood sugar without any dramatic symptoms. Jayne (1993) interviewed men and women who had had diabetes for 6 to 20 years. Women with family members affected by diabetes knew to seek medical help, but others did not.

For diabetics, medical professionals soon identified their problem with simple blood sugar tests. By contrast, women with multiple sclerosis (MS) had great difficulty obtaining a diagnosis. Diagnosis of MS may require at least two different attacks of symptoms in different parts of the nervous system, so even when physicians are considering MS a possibility, firm diagnosis can take months or years (Gregg et al., 1989, p. 245). In the meantime, these fluctuating symptoms, hard to document, are discounted. Many women with MS have been sent to mental health providers and given a diagnosis such as depression as the explanation for their symptoms (Klonoff & Landrine, 1997). Fitzgerald and Paterson (1995) interviewed Australian women with MS, one of whom thought she might be losing her mental faculties:

> For a while there when I did first get it and I didn't know that it was MS, I
> started thinking maybe I am imagining this, it is all up here, you know. (p.
> 15)

Fibromyalgia, a painful muscle disorder affecting mainly women, with symptoms like chronic flu, is usually diagnosed by excluding other causes of the symptoms. This involves prolonged and painful testing. Schaefer (1995) found that some women with this illness had spent up to 12 years with symptoms before being diagnosed. Like the woman with MS, many worried or were told that their problem was mental or emotional. They noticed something was wrong, that they had prolonged flulike symptoms, including muscle pain and extreme fatigue, and fearing the worst, began to try to convince others of the seriousness of their symptoms. After months or years of nonconfirmation, all the women felt as if they were breaking down, "losing their marbles." They depleted their financial, physical, psychological, and social resources in their efforts to manage daily life while searching for a name for their problem.

Finding out one's diagnosis often brings relief, even if it means facing serious limitations or early death, because at least it demonstrates that one had been correct in believing something was wrong. Having a diagnosis gives the ability to project into the future. Register (1987), herself living with a rare liver disease, interviewed a number of individuals with different chronic illnesses and found they all had a degree of relief when diagnosed: "I could have just hugged that doctor for taking me seriously and deciding to get to the bottom of this" (p. 13). Women wanted to be taken seriously when they reported symptoms, but this did not always occur. Cultural devaluing of women's perceptions of their own reality and their own self-doubt no doubt played a part in interactions with physicians and social contacts, further demoralizing women and isolating them from sources of support.

Once a diagnosis was made and symptoms were being addressed, women began the reckoning process, facing the personal and social ramifications of having a specific illness. While being diagnosed meant they now had a legitimate explanation for being unable to meet social or work obligations, it also brought grieving, as it meant loss of long life, the capacity to do their accustomed work or to participate in social and family life as they were used to, or the news that their symptoms would continue indefinitely. Grieving was a necessary step in reckoning with illness, as described by a woman with MS and rheumatoid arthritis:

> When you lose your health with a chronic illness, you've lost part of you,
> just as if you'd lost a husband or wife. . . . People . . . weren't giving me the
> time to mourn, to feel sorry for myself. . . . You have to go through the
> whole process, before you can come back and do or be whatever you can
> without that thing you've lost. (Register, 1987, p. 22-23)

This grieving could be delayed for years after diagnosis, if the initial presentation of the diagnosis by medical professionals was overly optimistic or if initial symptoms subsided. Grief thus could resurge as the illness flared up, bringing with it new meanings of loss. Chronic sorrow, a pervasive sadness that recurred when they were reminded of what illness had taken from them, was first described in bereaved parents but also was described by the majority of women with MS in one study (Hainsworth, 1994).

In accepting a diagnosis, women also must grasp and accept the expected trajectory of an illness as they understand it. For some diseases, there is a predictable course, and for others, it is completely uncertain. Some illnesses have ups and downs but remain at a generally steady level, whereas others involve inevitable decline and early death. A woman and her physician may have differing expectations of the illness trajectory based on what has been told to her and how she interprets the information in the face of her other experience. The trajectory of illness demands adjustments in one's current identity and the rewriting of one's anticipated future (Strauss, 1975). It may be revised as symptoms and the understanding of illness change over time. Women also may work on altering the illness trajectory by changing their attitudes and behavior.

Being a Naive Newcomer

Once diagnosed, many women with diabetes, multiple sclerosis, and fibromyalgia felt a desire to gather all available information about the illness to be able to predict their future course and make adjustments in their lives. Some were given simplistic or incomplete information about their diseases by medical professionals. Frustration was acute when women had been waiting for a diagnosis to give certainty and then found that little was known about their condition or, in the case of MS, that it had a very unpredictable course.

Even in the early phases of illness, women made judgments about the information they were given as being too complex or too simple, outdated or current, and overly frightening or reassuring and satisfying. When they perceived gaps between what they were told and what they needed in order to formulate the meaning of the illness for themselves, many went to libraries, talked to friends and family, contacted national foundations, and otherwise tried to bring themselves up to date. Those with less education or resources and those with stigmatizing diagnoses delayed asking questions until they found a knowledgeable person with whom they felt comfortable. They suffered alone with their disease and their uncertainty about its meaning.

As they interacted with health professionals, women examined both the content and the context of what they were told:

I can understand now their prejudices, because they're in a whole different

world than I was, and they had the knowledge and if they start talking to me
in their language, they figured I wouldn't know what they were talking about
anyway, so why even bother explaining to me. (Thorne, 1993, p. 31)

Some persons with chronic illness had little basis for judgment about what
they were told and relied on their medical caregivers. For example, women with
diabetes reported that the prevailing message given to them as new patients was
that if they dutifully measured their blood sugar and kept it within acceptable
ranges by following diet, exercise, and insulin regimens, they would be able to
enjoy an otherwise normal life.

Jayne (1993) found that during the initial period when new diabetics were
taught survival skills of how to manage self-testing, insulin administration, diet,
and managing high and low blood sugar, they were given verbal messages and
instructional materials extolling the potential of anyone with diabetes to lead a
normal, active life as long as they continued their self-care regimen.
Complications such as blindness, kidney failure, and heart disease were also
mentioned but as distant possibilities, in the context of what could happen if the
regimen was not adhered to.

Soon afterward, these patients found that diabetes required a distinctly
abnormal amount of self-denial and illness care tasks. Even with close attention
to self-care, blood sugar control was unreliable, and many adjustments were
needed to approximate stability. New diabetics were very dependent on medical
professionals to manage decisions about food, insulin doses, exercise, and daily
activities. Early on, when they became acutely ill, they sought to return to a
stricter version of the previous regime in hope of achieving the promised
normalcy. Only later did they come to realize that normalcy with diabetes had to
be redefined.

Similarly, Price (1993) interviewed men and women with diabetes who also
described an initial phase of trying out the prescribed regimen, following
instructions as carefully as possible with the belief that if they did so, their
blood sugar control would be stable and life could go on as before. However,
their regimens were found to be so restricting and time-consuming that they
sought to see whether small adjustments could be made without compromising
their health. "Cheating" on their diet was the first change made by all. They
closely monitored the effects of these little changes, and when little harmful
impact was perceived at the time, many progressed to other modifications of
their regime.

Newcomers to MS had even less understanding of what their diagnosis
meant for their futures because their doctors could not predict the course or
severity of the disease. Women faced a life of extreme uncertainty, as they were
told that this disease could come and go over time and could have only minor
effects or lead to complete disability or death. Some saw their life as a roller
coaster: "You don't know if it's going to be an up day, feeling good, or a down

day in which just getting out of bed is difficult." (Quinn, Barton, & Magilvy, 1995, p. 22). In the first year after diagnosis, women said that facing life with the unpredictability of MS required most of all maintaining a fighting spirit (p. 22) until more knowledge was gained about how the illness would affect them personally and how to cope with it.

These early months and years with chronic illness were an assault on the self: one's identity in the world, one's credibility, and one's projected biography for the future. Women struggled to understand and cope with their symptoms using what medical professionals had to offer. They tried to relate to others in ways that legitimated their illness but retained their former selfhood. They wondered about their future in work and home life and sought to learn what they could about their condition in moments of drive to overcome it. In moments of discouragement and despair, they grieved for the identity and hope they had once had.

Charmaz, in extensive research with the chronically ill (1980, 1983, 1991, 1995), found that loss of self was a fundamental form of suffering in chronic illness. Selfhood was lost due to restriction of movement and influence, social isolation, being discredited by others, and being a burden on others (1983). Ill persons found that being unable to comply with American values of hard work, independence, and individual responsibility made them feel extremely unworthy and unlikeable by themselves and others, yet during periods of suffering, they continued to believe that they were personally responsible for controlling the impact of illness in their lives.

Self-pity (Charmaz, 1980) could become immobilizing over time and cause sufferers to give up hope of improvement or effort to find reward in life. Self-pity could be reversed by improvement in physical status, affirmation by others, and motivation to change brought on by comparing oneself to less fortunate others or to one's former self. Some women decided that they were not going to let their burden of illness keep them from participating in life:

> I was sick of their pitying looks and concerned voices . . . but after a time I realized I pitied myself more than anyone else pitied me. So then and there I decided, I wouldn't let this keep me down; I was going to do something with the rest of my life. (p. 142)

In order to adapt to impairment, chronically ill persons had to experience and assess their impaired bodies and altered appearance, give in to the ongoing fluctuating presence of illness, and revise their identity goals (Charmaz, 1995). To surrender, individuals had to give up the culturally prescribed goals of victory over illness and control over the body. They had to work toward accepting that the impaired body was indeed part of the changing self.

Adjusting to Unpredictability

A central fact of chronic illness that many women reckoned with was that their health would remain unpredictable despite all their efforts and those of their doctors. Even when the initial diagnosis had brought a sense of certainty and relief, the reality of how illness affected them on a day-to-day basis turned out to be quite variable. Using their initial understandings, women with diabetes, for example, would dutifully make adjustments in their diet or insulin to address unexpected changes in blood sugar, but their efforts didn't have the same effect each time. They began to think about the long-term complications of the disease they had learned about in the beginning but had brushed aside. Would they become blind or develop kidney failure? Jayne (1993) noted that persons with diabetes felt betrayed when the initial messages of promised normalcy were proven false.

Diabetes required coming to grips with unrelenting vulnerability (Armstrong, 1987, 1990). Individuals felt acute personal accountability for the control of their disease, yet the burden of this responsibility was often too great. They craved a normal life in which they could eat spontaneously, travel at will, and not be burdened by self-testing, planned exercise, and calculations of food and insulin. Constant vigilance was too much for many to sustain indefinitely, and in periods of frustration they would "cheat" on their diets or monitoring and then "repent" afterwards with renewed efforts to establish healthy blood sugar levels. This frustration-cheat-repent cycle was a phase for some and a continuing pattern for others, as they struggled with the demands of their illness and their desires for the old version of normalcy.

Women with MS came to realize that their attacks could come on in the midst of an activity, making even simple chores unpredictable. Hainsworth (1986, 1994) interviewed women with MS who described a variety of surprising and sometimes dangerous sudden onsets of weakness:

> One time, I fell when I was talking to my neighbor on the telephone. (Hainsworth, 1986, p. 94)

> I fell just before I went into the hospital. . . . I walked outdoors and fell. I started to cry. I wasn't hurt, just disgusted. (p. 96)

A third woman described a time when she was peeling potatoes and became so weak that she couldn't finish the job. The women saw these incidents as not only annoying but frightening, as they implied future deterioration.

Fatigue was an unending problem of MS (Stuifbergen & Rogers, 1997). Fatigue led to emotional despair and inability to concentrate, as well as difficulty sustaining interactions: "Talking with people, you don't want the conversation to go on very long, just to finish as soon as possible" (p. 5). Perhaps most difficult was that fatigue was invisible, and a woman could appear completely well when she found it necessary to withdraw from social engagements or work responsibilities. Fatigue also was a significant problem for women with fibromyalgia.

Accepting the Ill-Person Identity

Grasping the Impact on the Self

To learn how to live with a disease, women needed first to accept that in the eyes of others and themselves, they indeed were affected with a health problem that would limit their freedom to choose activities or to anticipate longevity or sustained capability. Some women moved quickly to learn about their illness and integrate it into their identity, but others resisted this self-labeling or modified it to lessen its impact. In some situations, family or coworkers had difficulty accepting a woman's changed identity, especially if the illness did not produce visible change or impairment.

This work on one's identity required time, as at first the true impact of the illness was not known. It required experiencing the changed body and the demands of illness, internalizing social messages about the illness and the role of the ill person, and fitting this information into the "me" that had existed before the onset of illness (Corbin & Strauss, 1988). Over time, women were able to create a revised yet consistent sense of who they now had become, with some strengths and abilities intact but others lost or in jeopardy. Then, they could begin to demonstrate to themselves and others how their new selves would move forward on different life trajectories.

Intrusion of Illness Demands

Women had to learn by experience the degree of intrusion or burden of their illness demands. Diabetes was certainly burdensome. Blood sugar measurement and preparing and injecting insulin had to be done several times daily, and food had to be planned, measured, and prepared according to dietary guidelines. Sweets were to be avoided. Regular exercise was important to minimizing insulin needs and maintaining stable blood sugar. This all had to be fitted into schedules of work and family responsibilities. Women varied in the ease with which they incorporated these tasks into their daily lives. For some, it was much more intrusive than for others, depending on the meaning of these actions, the value placed on intangibles such as health and long life, and the resources available to help with this self-care.

Armstrong (1990) described diabetes's demands as "life-encompassing and constant" (p. 102). Not only did women have to perform many daily tasks related to blood sugar control, but they were expected to minimize risk of future complications by practicing meticulous skin care, minimizing stress and emotional upset that could upset blood sugars, managing symptoms of low blood sugar which could lead to coma, and responding to high blood sugar by calculating and experimenting with new insulin doses.

Meanwhile, there was usually no visible or noticeable effect of these preventive actions, making it easy to skip them or to challenge the belief that they made a difference at all. Women with diabetes learned the skills to manage all these burdens, but finding the motivation to do so was much more difficult. "I guess it gets back to either because I want to or don't want to" (Armstrong, 1990, p. 103). The demands of diabetes were especially difficult to accept day in and day out because motivation alone sustained these efforts rather than immediate evidence of success or failure.

Physically debilitating conditions, such as multiple sclerosis, had different demands. Fatigue was a constant issue. Simple processes--even getting up in the morning--had to be done differently. Daily tasks of using the bathroom and maintaining bladder control became troublesome for women with MS, and unexpected weak spells led women to take precautions such as carrying canes, not going out alone, or quitting jobs that were too dangerous or demanding. Monitoring themselves for signs of impending weak spells became a constant practice. If disability became more permanent, women with MS had to confront the identity-altering obstacles of depending on others and using wheelchairs, bladder control aids, devices to assist with feeding, and so forth (Hainsworth, 1986).

Exclusion From Normal Life

Perhaps the most difficult part of reckoning with chronic illness was discovering the degree to which the illness interfered with participating in family life and traditions, activities with others, recreation and spontaneous fun, and the feeling of being equal and worthy in social contexts. Women with diabetes reported that being normal to them was "eating what you want when you want it and includes liberal portions of desserts. Normal is staying healthy without exercising" (Armstrong, 1990). A regimented, illness-obsessed lifestyle does not feel ordinary or normal.

The demands of monitoring and medication isolated women with diabetes from others without such burdens. To add insult to injury, others could easily forget that a woman was subject to restrictions or even wittingly or unwittingly sabotage the woman's efforts:

I was at someone's house one night and they said we fixed this nice salad for you. It was so good . . . and she was very proud of herself, and I said, are you sure this doesn't have any sugar in it, and she said no. . . . It was so sweet and so good, and she gave me the recipe later and she put Karo syrup in it. (Armstrong, 1990, p. 105)

A woman who suffered an episode of low blood sugar while skiing described her difficulty in accepting her limits:

I kept falling and standing up, falling and standing up. The instructor came over and said, "Are you OK, should I get you a stretcher?" "I'm fine," I never told her a thing. I never knew what was happening. . . . My husband reacted with anger. . . . It took most of the afternoon [for me] to come around enough to get back to the hotel. When I came home, I said [to myself], "Yes, you can live a life like everybody else, but you do have to make changes to your life; you really have to admit that you are different." (Jayne, 1993, p. 134)

Likewise, women with physical disabilities or illnesses that restrict walking, driving, games, going out to movies or to visit friends, participating in family holiday dinners or preparing them, and the infinite other social interactions central to women's self-concepts suffer stigma, unfair exclusion, self-pity, and low self-esteem. In a culture that values physical strength, conquering physical pain and weakness to achieve independence, and using "mind over matter" to vanquish the obstacles of poor health, women whose illnesses preclude such valor feel less than worthy. This combined with the social isolation of being restricted to home or a small physically navigable territory may require total revamping of how responsibilities can be met and how work gets done: How do I buy and wrap birthday gifts? How do I get across the room to hug my daughter? How do I sell real estate or clean houses or program computers, when this is what I do for work, but my body won't let me?

Needing to Accept Help

The demands of illness that cause the most stress to many American women are those that create dependency on others or becoming a burden (Charmaz, 1980). Being unable to reciprocate is a very uncomfortable predicament when women are accustomed to a self-definition as one who gives to others rather than receives care. Accommodating others' help on a daily basis, while being unable to fill former duties in the household, demands readjustments in relationships, which can be positive or extremely stressful.

Some women with MS worried about strain on their husbands, who helped them bathe and dress each morning before going to work and then faced household chores when they returned each evening (Hainsworth, 1986). In some of these families, conflict was visible and acknowledged by partners; in others, it was harbored in mutual resentment. For a few, open communication and planning with spouses kept the stress at a manageable level. Although they needed help from their families and wanted it to be available without punishment or resistance, women did not want to be viewed as any more disabled than they actually were. Some refused to install ramps or obtain "handicapped" license plates, although this would have made their lives easier.

These women with MS demonstrated the dual burdens of their capricious physical condition: to defend and accommodate the reality of their physical limitations within the scope of home life, while hiding or minimizing these limitations in other social contexts. They sought respect for their disability at home and the illusion of ability outside the home. Sympathy and help were acceptable and sometimes essential from those close to them, but pity and devaluation were not tolerable from strangers. These double standards led to inconsistency in their behavior that puzzled and frustrated some family and friends (Hainsworth, 1986).

Exposing the Limits of Medical Wisdom

A final truth of chronic illness that women reckoned with was the inability of medical professionals to ease their burdens or restore normalcy. Jayne (1993) termed this realization "confronting the illusion of promised normality," and Thorne (1990, 1993) described it as "disenchantment." Over time, women realized that their doctors were not infallible or all knowing, and that the burden of understanding and solving the problems of their illness would fall on their own shoulders. Women's trust in their doctors was shaken when promised improvement or stability in their conditions did not occur (Jayne, 1993), when doctors reneged on agreements to provide certain treatments (Thorne, 1993), when doctors did not show personal caring in times of crisis, or when after a period of time it became clear to the woman that she knew better than the doctor how to manage the ups and downs of her condition.

Disenchantment with medical care brought intense feelings of isolation and self-doubt. Some women thought they were doing something wrong if their doctors would not or could not help them. Others felt betrayed by the medical system or angry at individual practitioners. For women who had been waiting months or years for a definitive diagnosis only to find that even then, there was little or no treatment available to alleviate the symptoms they were suffering, the prospect of going it alone without a secure medical structure to guide them was daunting.

In a culture in which medical knowledge and authority are highly esteemed, women who confronted the limits and failures of medicine wondered what stability remained. Some wondered if, given the lack of earthly help for them, they were being punished for their sins or unworthiness or were being abandoned by God (Hainsworth, 1986). Depression, despair, and abandoning the struggle were the initial outcome for some, whereas others allowed their illnesses to become their new identities and structures for living and allowed themselves to become dependent on the medical system despite its limits (Charmaz, 1995). Only gradually did women make their way toward a "guarded alliance" with medical personnel (Thorne, 1993).

RECONCILING: MAKING PEACE WITH THE UNINVITED GUEST

From Victim to Voyager: Refocusing the Meaning of Illness

As in cancer and heart disease, women made peace with their illnesses by making peace with their bodies. Only when the changed body became familiar, known, and accepted with its real limitations could adaptation to illness begin (Charmaz, 1995). To a certain degree, this involved objectifying the body, observing its changes as reflections of the illness process. But women also reaccepted their bodies as limited but necessary parts of themselves, the vehicles through which they must work toward a different life and self. To do this, they became attuned to and respectful of the demands of their bodies in new ways (Jayne, 1993).

Women reappraised their bodies, not only in light of what once was good but of what could be worse. Over time, the burden increased in both diabetes and MS. Diabetes became more difficult to manage for some women, as blood sugar changes began to occur with less warning (Callaghan & Williams, 1994), and MS could bring increasing weakness and debility. They continually reenvisioned their levels of functioning as the midpoint on a continuum--not totally dysfunctional, not fully functional, but at a reasonable midpoint. This flexible self-appraisal was revised as physical capability changed, to maintain the fortifying perspective of not being as badly off as one could be. For example, several women with MS accepted that they needed assistance with mobility but were grateful that they still had their vision (Hainsworth, 1986). Women with diabetes had come to grips with the fact that their illness was permanent with no respite from daily care, but in reconciling, they came to view this daily bodily obligation as less onerous than problems such as loss of consciousness due to an insulin reaction or long-term complications of blindness or limb amputations (Armstrong, 1990).

Close relationships were challenging for women whose bodies demanded constant attention. The illness became like a third party in a marriage or partnership. Register (1987) found that even women who otherwise were well-adapted to their illnesses struggled periodically to accept their less-than-perfect bodies when intimacy was involved. A woman who wore an ostomy bag after intestinal surgery told her,

> I couldn't ever imagining myself attracting somebody in a bikini or in any of those normal, stereotypical ways. . . . If I was to develop any kind of intimate relationship with anybody, that was going to have to be dealt with. . . . It was like having someone say "OK, all your usual ways of relating to people have to be completely changed." (p. 38-39)

Sexual intimacy was extremely difficult when unpredictability, pain, or disfigurement detracted from women's comfort in their bodies. Some women with diabetes endured chronic vaginal infections that made sex very painful and made them worry about vaginal odor (LeMone, 1993). Couples in long-term relationships were sometimes able to adapt by finding other ways of expressing affection and being intimate, but unpartnered women faced great challenges, struggling to maintain a feeling of attractiveness and worth as a potential intimate partner.

Women who continued some degree of athletics or physical activity despite chronic illness felt better about their bodies than did women who were prevented from doing so by immobility or did not have these skills to fall back on. Affirmation from others was central to regaining a sense of bodily worth, and husbands played critical roles in this. In general, younger women seemed more distressed than did older women by changes in physical appearance, as they faced the most dramatic violations of personal and social expectations (Charmaz, 1995).

Re-Valuing the Self: Editing the Autobiography

Just as they reconnected, with new respect, with their newly separate, changing bodies, women who reconciled with their chronic illnesses had to find a way to accept and value themselves. They rediscovered their traits and unique abilities that had survived the onset of illness and used these persisting qualities as foundations. Paradoxically, the illness was both part of the self and distinct from it. Register (1987) described the importance to herself of separating what her diseased liver did and what the self did. When her doctor told her, "You're febrile again," she reframed it for him as, "The fever is back" (p. 42). She called this a mind game: knowing that her identity included a chronic illness yet not letting it become the definition of who she was.

When Register (1987) asked a variety of chronically ill people whether they thought of themselves as ill, she obtained a variety of reactions. The seriousness of the external disease did not determine the identity as ill; rather, it was the degree to which the illness interfered with functions and roles they valued. One individual responded that she had an illness but did not think of herself as "sick" because she had no health problems other than MS (p. 45). Sometimes, the illness dominated the moment and the healthy self was in the background, determinedly working to prevail again. Then, when the illness was on course and more stable, women could view themselves as mostly healthy, while not denying the fragility of that health. They evolved a way of looking at themselves that maintained a sense of unity, in which a healthy consciousness could respond to and even devote itself fully to an ailing body without being overwhelmed by it (Charmaz, 1995). This unity of body and identity was most strained in times of unexpected suffering, when women were forced to expand their self-definition yet again to encompass a new symptom, threat, or limitation. Nevertheless, the self persisted, overshadowed at times by new burdens but rising again to reappraise the situation and redefine how a valued past identity could be retained despite suffering and loss.

Finding a Social Persona

Charmaz (1995) described reappraisal of self with illness as raising or lowering identity goals. Each person worked out a hierarchy of possible identities ranging from desired to undesirable, and adapted to their changing capacities by continually resetting their sights on the identities that seemed feasible and achievable. This adjustment over time enabled the chronically ill to continue to feel successful and useful, even when previous careers or roles were out of reach.

Identity shifts were worked out in the context of significant others' views and wishes (Charmaz, 1995, p. 669). Beyond intimate friends and family, the chronically ill faced other social contexts of work, casual acquaintances, public spaces, and so forth. With a growing understanding of the revised identities that had been shaped in their intimate social spheres, they were able to navigate outside those arenas with a sense of internal worth despite social approbation. Young chronically ill women faced the largest challenges (Charmaz, 1995). Partners of younger women were more tentative in their support of their ill wives and less likely to take over tasks than were husbands in older couples, where loyalty and attachment was well-established and perhaps less dependent on physical attractiveness or capability. Thus, younger women not only faced a greater burden of loss of physical attractiveness and desirability but were more often denied help and validation from current partners.

Even in caring and supportive relationships, conflicts arose in partners' views of women's appropriate identity goals. For example, a wife's valued work or volunteer role might be viewed by a husband as inappropriately tiring or stressful. Identity trade-offs were a means of retaining one valued role while giving up another one; for example, a professor might continue to write books but give up teaching. After such a trade-off, ill persons sought to redefine their choices in positive ways to minimize the loss (Charmaz, 1995, p. 671).

Register (1987) described an "etiquette of chronic illness" that women developed to deal with casual social situations. When colleagues asked, "How are you?" individuals were forced to make judgments about whether the asker really wanted to know, was simply making small talk, or was trying to determine whether the conversation could proceed. Second-guessing became part of daily interactions. One woman had determined over time that the best course was to spare others of her suffering:

> I'd say, "Oh, good." I don't really feel good. This is good compared to last week. . . . I don't want you to carry that image of me as always being sick. (Register, 1987, p. 49)

Another woman had developed a pattern of saying she was "all right" when her illness was continuing as usual and "terrific" when she felt really well. Likewise, she sought not to impose her difficulties on others and protect her privacy while keeping some shred of truth in her replies. Jayne (1993) described diabetics' disclosures as "selective transparency" (p. 147). Disclosure could bring help and support, such as during dangerous insulin reactions, but it also could bring unwanted stigma and possible threats to job security.

These strategies were ways of maintaining a social identity as healthy or as "having an illness" but managing well. Both of these were more honorable than "being ill" and needing help or sympathy. Yet, the cost of fending off inquiries was a nagging sense of isolation and dishonesty, coupled with dismay that even when others knew of their problems and asked in caring ways, an ill person was being brought back to the reality of the illness rather than being permitted to focus on other more rewarding parts of life (Register, 1987).

Friendships became delicate and ambiguous in the context of chronic illness. Women with illness feared slipping into constant dependency on friends' caring and good will, losing the mutuality and reciprocity that was possible during healthier times (Register, 1987). Illness could serve as a bond of intimacy but also as a barrier. Women described how they needed to demonstrate that their basic personalities had not changed--that they could laugh at themselves or continue to focus on life outside of illness--before friends regained their comfort with them.

The help available from friends could be practical or intangible, constant or unreliable. Part of the art of learning to live with chronic illness was learning to understand when friends were unable to help. Some women preferred not to involve their friends when their illnesses took turns for the worse, choosing to be alone and maintain self-respect rather than display their struggles and unattractiveness at these times. Others found that friends' presence enabled them to feel supported and loved in times of difficulty. Trustworthiness more than helpfulness was a central criterion for involvement of friends in one's illness over time. Friends were most valued who kept their word about promised help and who maintained respect and understanding while being honest when they were uncomfortable or confused. They would not silently become burdened and resentful of the ill woman's needs. When this balance was achieved in friendships, they enabled women to remain alive in the world in valued ways, as persons with history behind them and contributions to make rather than as needy victims seeking unending support (Register, 1987).

Taking Back the Reins: Personalizing Illness Management

Making Treatment Decisions

Part of shaping the trajectory of illness to suit one's identity needs is making decisions that move the trajectory in a direction compatible with one's own identity and preferred future. Kelly-Powell (1994) interviewed men and women with heart disease, kidney failure, or cancer shortly after they had made important treatment decisions. She found that these individuals did not base their treatment decisions on medical odds of success or recovery. Instead, they made "decisions of the heart" that fit with their past experience, their present life situation, and their expected future life context. When they were not given adequate information or were blocked from using these priorities to make treatment decisions, frustration resulted.

For example, a woman with kidney failure was receiving hemodialysis, which required going to a center for several hours several days a week. She wanted to return to continuous ambulatory peritoneal dialysis (CAPD), which is done at home by the woman herself several times a day by putting fluid through a catheter into the abdomen. She valued flexibility and being able to travel:

> I would much prefer to be on peritoneal dialysis than this. It gives me more freedom. . . . I had more independence. I could lead more of a normal life (Kelly-Powell, 1994, p. 116).

By contrast, another woman who taught children at her church wanted to maintain her outward appearance as much as possible. She rejected CAPD as a treatment option for her kidney failure because it involved bulky equipment worn on the abdomen under her clothing. For her, normal life meant not having to feel self-conscious in front of a group, and she opted for hemodialysis.

The patients made their choices based on religious faith, love and support from their families that made them feel responsible to keep going in treatment, their levels of trust in health care providers, and their personal and cultural values and beliefs. One African American woman noted,

> For black people, we've always been taught that you're born with that's what you're gonna die with. . . . We feel as if God has given us that, that's what we need to go to the grave with. (Kelly-Powell, 1994, p. 97)

She was facing kidney failure, but accepting someone else's kidney did not feel right to her, although it would have brought improvement in her quality of life. These individuals made their choices based on the best fit with their identities, habits, family constellation, and beliefs about the world, and only used the statistics given them by their doctors to give legitimacy to their decisions.

Adjusting and Inventing Self-Care

To reconcile their ongoing lives and commitments with the demands of chronic illness, many women abandoned earlier notions of reliance on health care providers for solutions to daily problems and fluctuations and developed their own approaches and routines. Women with MS called this becoming one's own doctor, keeping the physician posted but forming one's own opinions about the best course of action (Hainsworth, 1994).

Women with diabetes, both in Sweden (Ternulf Nyhlin, 1991) and the United States (Jayne, 1993; Price, 1993), found that they had to alter or abandon prescribed regimens when they did not produce optimal blood sugar control or were not workable within the context of their lives. Ternulf Nylin (1991) described the tenuous balance of illness demands and other areas of life and relationships as "walking a fine line" (p. 187). Jayne termed this level of control "pragmatic sufficiency" (p.141); Price (1993) noted that individuals developed a self-management style that "works for me" (p. 37). This might involve strict or less stringent control of blood sugar. The fit with the individual's personality, life context, and understanding of the implications of the illness determined their pattern of self-care.

> It always struck me that it would be great if all diabetics were . . . very pragmatic, highly organized, lived very disciplined lives, and loved schedules. Unfortunately, I think God has a sense of humor, at least in my case. And he certainly married me to the wrong disease. . . . The hardest thing in the world for me is to try to be very systematic and orderly in my existence. (Jayne, 1993, p. 133)

The ups and downs of blood sugar variations affected every aspect of everyday life, a reality that women with diabetes learned the hard way. Significantly, persons with diabetes were more likely to alter their regimens than their life priorities, although both were modified in response to the illness (Jayne, 1993). For example, one individual let her blood sugar run higher than medically desirable when she was out at social events, to avoid the embarrassment of an insulin reaction with its perspiration, anxiety, mood changes, and possible loss of consciousness.

When they had discovered the limits of their health care providers' knowledge and insight, many persons with MS, diabetes, and fibromyalgia took their regimens into their own hands. Women with diabetes learned over time which bodily symptoms were indicative of blood sugar shifts, how to give the amounts of insulin that would compensate for the shifts without overcompensating, how to manage food planning in the context of their other activities, and when they needed to consult medical professionals. Gradually, this informal monitoring became as or more important than the blood testing they had been taught:

> The technology started me off, so I would know what my body was telling me, then I guess I sort of dropped the technology and [was] just going with the body. . . . Occasionally I'll go to the technology for a specific reason. [When] I'm getting a few signals from my body . . . I'll check with technology. (Jayne, 1993, p. 125)

Thorne (1990) coined the phrase "constructive noncompliance" to describe chronically ill persons' deviations from medical prescriptions when they followed their own judgment without severing health care relationships. Chronically ill persons juggled recommendations from a variety of professionals, sorting through the different information until they developed a synthesis that made sense within their own experience. When they disregarded medical advice, it was a conscious and reasoned decision rather than an ignorant or willful rebellion. They personalized their use of information, did not follow advice they believed erroneous or harmful, yet did not confront their physicians, to maintain ties to them in case of future need. In choosing not to follow professional advice, these individuals were taking responsibility for their own illness management, a role they felt prepared to fill.

Becoming Accountable to the Self

As women discovered the benefits of customized self-care, they also shouldered the responsibility for its burdens. No longer could the illness be viewed as a temporary aberration or a problem in the hands of medical professionals. Diabetics in particular had to take on "food accountability" (Jayne, 1993, p. 152), a constant struggle between the desire for unrestricted access to favorite foods and their responsibility to manage food's power to disrupt blood sugar control and increase risk of later complications. Constant planning, surveillance, and decision making about what and when to eat took away much of the pleasure in food. Some persons with diabetes made allowances for themselves; they sought to maintain some degree of normalcy in their eating to balance their need for autonomy with the impositions of their illness:

> I have to take in all these factors and find the way to balance them. . . . All I can do is the best I can do, and that includes allowing myself to have the forbidden foods. (p. 154)

Women with childhood experiences of eating disorders and emotional trauma had a particularly hard time being honest with themselves and accountable for their food intake. Yet when life events revealed to them the value of their own survival, some sought counseling and peer support to reclaim some control over their lives and their illness management. Armstrong (1990) also noted that to become accountable for self-care, diabetics had to reach a turning point in which an untoward event made them newly aware of their vulnerability to complications. Then, they moved forward to reconcile with the demands of their illnesses and reap the newly valued benefits of health and increased self-respect.

Becoming an Expert

Women who worked on becoming reconciled to chronic illness became highly knowledgeable about their conditions, often more knowledgeable than their doctors. They gained this knowledge through evaluation of a wide variety of information sources and testing of the information in their own experience. In becoming expert, women learned when they could manage their own illness and when outside help was needed.

Persons with diabetes not only took responsibility for their care but for gathering the most relevant knowledge available and then taking the initiative to apply it to their own lives. The novice person with diabetes made laborious calculations of food, blood sugar, and insulin, whereas the expert developed a fluid awareness of what to do (Ternulf Nyhlin, 1991). They combined expert physical awareness of the body's messages with expert scientific awareness of the mechanisms of their illness.

Using the System

With deep and valid understandings of their illnesses, women were better able to advocate for their needs within medical care systems, even when this involved requesting special exceptions to medical protocol. Register (1987) described learning from experience that she was able to identify signs of impending infection, and she would request antibiotic treatment even before the infection could be detected by standard tests. Early efforts to ignore her feelings of impending trouble and be a good patient brought painful and dangerous delays of treatment, so she learned to negotiate around doctors' doubt of her knowledge, taking upon herself the responsibility for the consequences. "We simply wanted to protect ourselves against a familiar form of suffering, and that meant sharing responsibility for diagnosis and treatment" (p. 202).

Women developed deep understandings not only of their own illnesses but of the medical care system in which they sought care. They learned whom to talk to to get things done, how long they could expect to wait for action, and which delays were reasonable and which were unreasonable. They became patient in another sense of the word: capable of tolerating delay, discomfort, and their ongoing burden of illness with calm and equanimity. Yet, in return they looked for reasonable accommodation and collaboration from health professionals (Register, 1987).

Once patients' naive trust in their health care system had been betrayed, they worked to reconstruct a new kind of limited and self-protecting relationship (Thorne, 1993). Thorne described four patterns of reconstructed trust. In "hero worship," patients who had low confidence in themselves singled out one professional as eminently trustworthy, although others were not expected to be reliable. In "resignation," patients with neither self-confidence nor trust in their professionals continued on in unsatisfactory health care relationships in case the relationship might be useful at some point in the future. "Consumerism" occurred when the patient had a high degree of confidence in herself and little trust in the system, which they sought to use to their own best advantage. Last, "team playing" was the most reciprocal form of reconstructed trust, in which confident individuals collaborated with certain health care professionals perceived as trustworthy and understanding of their personal goals.

Clearly, as women develop confidence in their own self-knowledge, they fare better in health care interactions. Being heard, believed and valued were critical components of developing a balanced trusting relationship with a health professional (Register, 1987). Women who felt their symptoms were being viewed as potentially important and biologically based rather than as psychosomatic were much more likely to bond with their doctors and follow their advice.

Finding Peers

Role models were invaluable in reconciling to chronic illness. It was reassuring and inspiring just to know that someone else was facing similar burdens and finding ways to go on building a life. Meeting others with long-term experience could help newly diagnosed illness sufferers look ahead and project the impact of illness on their own futures. Although it was important to see the reality of possible future decline as it occurred in others' lives, women interpreted others' experience in light of their own personalities, histories, and resources. They used the evidence selectively in working out personal strategies for overcoming obstacles (Register, 1987). These peer encounters had an additional potential benefit. When peers shared the same illness, the illness became "normal" in that context. Women's individuality and social identities could then be appreciated more fully. For example, they became "the artist" or "the newlywed" or "the lawyer" rather than "the woman with MS."

Same-illness groups were a mixed blessing for individuals still working on reconciling their lives with their illnesses. Some resisted joining self-help groups for fear that the illness would become the main component of their identities (Register, 1987). They avoided being associated with a "subculture" that would overtake their identities and make more difficult the task of confining the influence of illness in their lives.

Women generally were comfortable with others who accommodated the demands of illness to the degree that they themselves hoped to accommodate them. In this sense, they sought role models for reconciling, looking for persons like themselves who had done this before. For example, a woman who was reluctant to start exercising to control her diabetes would probably not seek out a fellow diabetic who effortlessly maintained an exercise regimen and had always been active. She might seek comfort in knowing a peer who was sedentary yet claimed no ill effects. If she experienced a negative consequence of her inactivity; then she would be likely to look for a woman who had managed to begin exercising for the first time late in life. Role models thus can provide road maps for accommodating illness demands.

Reinventing "Normal"

When women successfully integrate chronic illness into their lives, they make the most of what may be a diminished scope of activity and capacity for participation in the world, learn to face uncertainty as an everyday state, and find ways of minimizing the threats their illness poses to what they hold most dear, including life itself. As Charmaz (1991) noted, life with chronic illness consists of an endless series of good days and bad days. Yet, with a sense that the illness has meaning and limits, and with self-efficacy to manage illness's impact on their lives and futures, women can come to see their existence as normal even when it has little resemblance to most others' lives. Normalizing can perhaps best be described as finding a balance between demands and comforts using internal and external resources, while nurturing the unique and growing self that is beyond the illness.

Submitting to Self-Regulation

Normal life with chronic illness requires maintaining awareness of the bodily changes that signal shifts in the illness process and responding rapidly to changes that may signal a turn for the worse. In addition, women must plan ahead for the unexpected, as when women with MS bring a companion or a walker when shopping in case a weak spell comes on suddenly or when women with diabetes bring food on an airplane in case the meal does not come in time to prevent an insulin reaction.

Self-regulation requires intimate awareness of the body's illness behavior, as learned over months and years with the disease. It also demands self-discipline, motivated by a deep understanding that without denying oneself some spontaneity and pleasure, the self will not be able to continue. Last, self-regulation requires work, completing many tasks over the course of the day to accommodate to the illness and keep it from veering out of control. It may include restraining oneself from participating in vigorous activities that will bring on increased weakness. It requires controlling emotional responses to one's own incapacity and others' misunderstanding, pity, denigration, and disbelief.

This emotional self-monitoring is part of normal life for women with fibromyalgia, chronic pain, and many other conditions in which emotional upset worsens the physical symptoms of illness. Personal experience over time and the ability to learn from new events seem to be the only way to learn how to handle the unexpected. Getting through these predicaments once enables one to have the confidence to navigate through future contingencies.

This is not to say that all women with chronic illness who have normalized their lives maintain perfect control over themselves and their illnesses at all times. Each woman determines a "good-enough" level of self-regulation (Armstrong, 1990; Price, 1993; Ternulf Nyhlin, 1991) or pragmatic sufficiency (Jayne, 1993), in which she feels she is doing what she can to minimize the threats of worsening disease while still retaining self-determination. The outcome may not be exemplary illness management but rather a sense of controlling the impact of the illness to protect one's identity and other priorities in life.

Learning to Live With It

The emotional and cognitive sides of life with chronic illness require constant attention and nurturing. "Living day by day" was described by women with fibromyalgia (Schaefer, 1995) and reflects the importance of focusing on one day at a time to avoid becoming psychologically overwhelmed by pain, disability, loss, or fear of death. Living day by day also expresses the value of appreciating each day as it comes, counting one's blessings if only to keep from despairing over one's misfortunes. A sense of coherence despite fibromyalgia brought well-being, hope, self-worth, and freedom (Soderberg, Lundman, & Norberg, 1997). Women with MS described the importance of having a positive outlook, allowing time for feelings, staying happy, and avoiding self-blame (Hainsworth, 1994).

Being at peace with chronic illness does not mean feeling peaceful all the time. As did women with MS, Register (1987) described the importance of authentic emotional expression of suffering to cling to and validate the self. She found herself talking to her pain, begging it to spare her (p. 231). Indeed, women can relate to their illnesses as annoying, sneaky, and ever-present companions. In this way, the illness is kept at bay, and the self is strengthened against it while realizing that the illness is in fact part of the larger "me." In times of relief of suffering come floods of relief, gratitude, and hope. Illness is an emotional as well as a physical roller-coaster. Women who are adept at riding it learn when to restrain their emotional expression to prevent physical disruption, and when to let out feelings to maintain an integrated self.

> It was just one of those things that happens in life, but I wanted to do what I wanted to do when I wanted to do it, and I couldn't. I pounded my knees and said, "I'm going to fight this." (Register, 1987, p. 247)

Keeping active in and outside the house and reintegrating with life outside the home (Westra, 1991, 1993) are essential to self-continuity in normalizing chronic illness. Women who can maintain contact with the activities in the world that matter to them, whether by actively participating, communicating by letter or phone, or by simply watching out the window, are able to set illness aside momentarily and nurture parts of themselves that are alive and growing. During times of worsening illness, women may draw back to conserve strength for illness management, but selfhood and hope is strengthened when women can be employed outside the home or contribute to some social project, adapting their contribution according to their changing ability, and continue to maintain friendships and intimate relationships that adjust to but are not dominated by the illness (Register, 1987). Having a pet, a role in work or home that contributes to others' well-being, or a relationship, whether with a grandchild who visits or a spouse who appreciates words of love and appreciation, enables even seriously ill women to escape from their burden of dependency and isolation and remember that they are valuable contributors, deficits and all.

Women can find faith and inspiration in others' lives and the natural world, adding to their understanding of the meanings of their illnesses and the nature of their relationships with the world around them. This advice came from a woman with fibromyalgia:

> I do everything I always did. If I'm not feeling well, it may take me longer to

do things. What used to take me half an hour to clean, may take me an hour.
I love to walk and hike. I just take a cane with me. . . .. I have the attitude that
I must make do, I must go on. I don't let it get to me. (Schaefer, 1995, p.
100)

For women with MS or other progressive diseases, as Charmaz (1995)
noted, it eventually became essential to accept the power of the illness and learn
to ride its ups and downs, rather than refusing to let go of any activities. What
remains constant, however, is the attitude of confidence that there is a way to
satisfy many of one's desires one way or another. Denying the demands of the
illness leads to lack of attention to essential needs. Accommodating to them
enables honest self-appraisal and constructive planning.

Women who adapt to illness constantly reappraise their situations, remind
themselves that they are better off than they might be, and work on accepting
their illness as part of who they are. This "counting one's blessings" was seen in
every study of successful adaptation to illness. "At least I'm not . . ." became a
way of reframing life with illness as better than some alternatives, and finding
something to be thankful for.

Seeing the Big Picture

Faith and religious practice were a source of comfort and understanding for
many women. Even if their faith traditions did not offer a helpful explanation of
illness, simply joining with others in prayer brought some serenity. Many who
had been sorely tested by illness found that spirituality emerged on its own as a
growing source of comfort, regardless of previous religious observance:

The sicker I got the more I turned to God . . . it has slowly evolved into
something more and more important: more faith than religion. (Register,
1987, p. 260)

Faith came not always from a structured religion but often from a deep
personal sense of coherence and purpose in life, discovered over time. Those
comforted by faith shared a belief that things would work out for the best and
that even when suffering was acute, somehow there would be a way through it.

When early death seemed likely, women pondered what would happen after
death and weighed the teachings of their religious traditions. This area was a
focus of continued searching for many living with illness, as they sought to
assemble a personal understanding that seemed both real and comforting.

Building and Giving Support

Women who successfully cope with chronic illness not only assemble and maintain a network that provides a variety of kinds of support but often find ways to help others. Parents, siblings, spouses, and children all make potential contributions to the well-being of women with chronic illnesses, yet each relationship brings potential burdens as well. Parents, for example, may be able to offer wisdom, love, financial support, and perhaps physical care, but their support also may create feelings of childishness, dependency, disempowerment, and accompanying depression. Spouses may offer intimate companionship, task-sharing, financial support, and sustenance of the life of the couple beyond illness, but spouses may also foster feelings of anger, helplessness, and guilt.

There are pitfalls to be avoided in any support relationship. Honest, respectful, and loving communication within relationships is essential, but even more important is maximizing the woman's contribution to that relationship, to reduce the feelings of burden, worthlessness, and dependency. Her contribution may be as little as saying thank you, or it may be extending herself to and beyond her limits at times to be able to give back. The strain of illness on relationships must be acknowledged and planned around. Honest self-appraisal by loved ones and the woman herself is needed if each person's ability to participate in a relationship is to be accurately assessed. Health care providers become close acquaintances for some women, whereas for others, distance from health professionals feels more comfortable between times of crisis. The goal for awoman with chronic illness is the development over time of a network of supporters who can meet her variety of support needs, including physical help; task-oriented work; financial survival; practical problem solving; emotional affection; empathy and insight; and knowledge of the illness and can also provide validation and a sense of worth.

Getting Stuck: When the Mountain is too Steep

Times come when a woman can feel no pride, fearlessness, or inner strength. The power of chronic illness to frustrate simple and complex goals is unending, and not all women have been granted the resources in their own histories, families, households, or economic situations with which to adapt to unending burden and uncertainty. As will be shown in the next chapter, pain and immobility are particularly wearing and disheartening.

Women can be stuck at the points of reckoning or reconciling. Reckoning, taking stock of the full impact of the illness, requires time and fortitude. We have all encountered ill individuals who seem stubbornly to refuse to accept their limitations. They may in fact have accepted them and moved on. The woman may be fully aware of her condition but unwilling to show weakness to others, as this woman with temporomandibular joint syndrome described:

> I try not to let people know of my problems outside of my home. I don't tell
> them all the pains I have, I try to keep it to myself. (Fitzgerald & Paterson,
> 1995, p. 17)

Or she may be feel most comfortable keeping her illness from her own
awareness on a daily basis, as described by the woman with fibromyalgia who
said, "I must go on. I don't let it get to me" (Schaefer, 1995, p. 100).
When the personal meaning of an illness is unacceptable or
incomprehensible, one can become stuck in reckoning. Until a woman works
out an understanding of why her illness happened, even if only to come to accept
that there is no explanation, she has difficulty moving toward adapting to the
illness and communicating her status to others. This adjustment must occur at
each new setback or loss of function:

> I used to laugh and joke about my MS, but when my eyesight went, it blew
> me . . .. I became very depressed, and the social worker from the MS Society
> told me that I was having a delayed grief reaction to my diagnosis.
> (Hainsworth, 1986, p. 94)

In fact, the meaning of the diagnosis changes with each new development.
Women can have accepted one level of disability or the possibility of becoming
worse but have difficulty when they experience subsequent changes and new
levels of dependence.

Grief may be expected and recurrent, but depression is not a necessary phase.
However, depression is a common "stuck" place in chronic illness, affecting a
large proportion of the acutely and chronically ill. If unrecognized, it can lead to
declining health and additional problems. Depressed patients have longer hospital
stays, participate less often and less fully in rehabilitation, and are less likely to
return to work and their previous level of functioning (Taylor & Aspinwall,
1990). If depression symptoms are confused with the physical effects of chronic
illness, or if depression is considered a normal reaction to severe illness, many
women may not be referred for mental health treatment.

Family members also can become stuck when they are unable to reckon
with the illness. The spouse of this woman with diabetes was ungenerous about
the physical changes in her body, and his complaints made her feel less
affectionate toward him and made sex more challenging:

> He always starts in that my breath stinks. He says it never used to stink
> before you were diabetic. I can brush my teeth, use mouthwash right before I
> go to bed, and he is still telling me I have to get a breath mint. As soon as
> he says that it's like everything I have built up sexually just plummets. I
> could care less what we do from that point on. (LeMone, 1993, p. 103)

One woman with MS lived with her mother, who was unwilling to install a wheelchair ramp at their home because it would announce to the world that her daughter's illness was progressive and permanent.

> My mother cannot accept my disease. She never went to an MS meeting to try to find out about it. If I get sick and stay in bed for a day, it bothers her. She says, "Why? Why? I am old, it should have been me." I went to a Cleveland Clinic and my mother thought they would give a pill and that would end my MS. She is looking for a miracle and says that God knows who to give this to. (Hainsworth, 1986, p. 59).

Even neighbors can cause pain to the ill person by questioning the legitimacy of the disability, as this woman with MS reported:

> When I first got ill, my next-door neighbor said that I was putting it all on so I wouldn't have to work. (Hainsworth, 1986, p. 66)

These ungenerous responses add to the burden of a woman's daily life with her illness, shaking self-esteem and increasing obstacles to reckoning.

Sometimes, women who have accepted the sad facts of illness still have difficulty reconciling with it or making a place in their lives for its demands and restrictions. This may be due to lack of knowledge about assistive devices or other tools or techniques or to lack of financial resources or helpers. Or they may be going through a process of trial and error, determining over time where changes are needed and where they can continue their prior activities. The uncertainty of chronic illness often makes it impossible to plan for all the accommodations that are needed. Women can become immobilized by uncertainty, the inability to anticipate how they will feel or function from day to day. Perhaps the largest challenge, however, is accepting on a deep level that the illness is part of their identities and then rebuilding self-congruent lives around it. Sorting through and redefining identity and priorities is a continuous and sometimes painful struggle.

HELPING WOMEN WITH CHRONIC ILLNESS

Personal Meanings

The most foundational area of work with women suffering chronic illness is helping them elicit, confront, and perhaps alter the personal meanings of the illness. This will involve uncovering women's medical knowledge, their cultural stereotypes and their social knowledge of the illness through family and friends, the spiritual or religious meanings of the illness, and their overall understanding of what caused it and what can be done about it. These meanings may not be foremost in women's priorities as they seek help. Dealing with family impact or daily living may bring women to counseling, or they may come for help accepting a turn for the worse after years of managing with a lesser degree of the same affliction.

Women who are suffering acutely have stated that simply providing empathetic listening is a valuable first step and not to be underrated, although women with MS reported that professionals and family were less likely than friends to provide empathy (Hainsworth, 1994). Then, probing gently for the meanings underneath the distress--the sources of pain and fear--can provide an initial "to-do list" for examining and dealing with the different origins of emotional pain. Many sessions may be occupied with simple ventilation of grief. This may be the most useful function of counseling for women with the personal and family resources to handle the other more mundane challenges of their illness.

Although these issues can be dealt with from many theoretical orientations, self theory and existential approaches offer some useful foci for confronting life-threatening illness. Basic questions--"Why me?" "Is this life worth living?" "What degree of choice do I have in this?"--will need to be addressed by many women. Remembering that acute fear arises from perceptions of meaninglessness and isolation and that being aware of and true to one's authentic self brings peace and integration, counselors can help women focus on who they are as unique individuals, how the illness threatens their special qualities and priorities, and how self-worth can be nurtured despite loss of previous outlets for self-expression.

Encountering and sustaining the healthy self becomes the ongoing goal of counseling work with chronically ill women over time. Counselors can use their presence and nonjudgmental acceptance to develop and maintain women's awareness of their enduring value despite physical losses. Exploration of ways of expressing this value can lead to planning for positive adaptation in many areas of women's lives.

Modifying Outlook and Viewpoint

There is increasing evidence for psychological contributions not only to the successful adjustment to illness but to its initial development. Negative affective style, anxiety, depression, and hostility, have been linked to heart disease, asthma, ulcers, and arthritis. Type A behavior, particularly its hostility, was first linked to heart attacks and now is known to include increased physical reactivity to stress--these individuals' pulse, blood pressure, and hormones increase rapidly, which may in turn create physical damage. Some researchers have suggested that a repressed, acquiescent personality may be a risk factor for cancer. A disease-prone personality has been described, but whether it directly causes illness or leads to unhealthy behaviors has yet to be discovered.

It is known, however, that positive outlook and emotional state, including optimism and perceived control or self-efficacy, has a potentially protective role against disease and improve recovery from illness (Taylor & Aspinwall, 1990). With these connections in mind, counselors can focus on women's habitual responses to stress and negative events and work on attitudinal and behavioral change. This kind of work must not be perceived by the client as punitive (implying that she caused her own illness) but rather should be presented as choosing a new perspective and taking charge of managing the impact of illness.

Health-promoting behaviors can be predicted by one's belief that the threat to health is severe, that a certain outlook or action will reduce the risk, and that one is capable of making the change. Strong intention to perform the healthy behavior is also a requirement for change. Using cognitive-behavioral interventions, counselors can work on each of these elements--believing that the threat of not responding to illness is serious, that the action will work, and that one can make the change. Then, the change can be planned and carried out. Relapse prevention techniques like those used to maintain smoking cessation can be used to reinforce success, once a change has been made. As part of learning self-monitoring and self-management, women can become sensitive to situations where social anxiety triggers negative self-appraisals and unhealthy behaviors. Counselors can teach relaxation techniques or assertiveness to provide tools for use in stressful situations (Taylor & Aspinwall, 1990).

Depression may be a stubborn problem as women struggle to face the personal meaning of disease. Counselors can work with women to help them take depression seriously, discriminate among symptoms, and seek treatment and medication when appropriate. This can be framed in a positive attitude of removing obstacles to health rather than as admitting weakness or failure. Active strategies, such as visualization, coping skills and relaxation training, and simple physical exercise "prescriptions" can combat depression and have been found more effective than support groups for severely depressed cancer patients (Telch & Telch, 1986). Achieving a change in one arena, even if only learning a new skill such as visualization, increases confidence that one can make changes in other areas of life.

Family and Relationships

Another major area of work for chronically ill women is the impact of illness on their ties to significant others. Whether counseling is pursued individually or with couples or family groups, the meanings of the illness to the family members must be elicited. These meanings may be very different than the woman's own views. Bringing out family members' stories of others they have known with the illness can uncover their beliefs and expectations. Medical information may be needed by family members who seem to misunderstand the effects of a disease, and families often must work on accepting the limits of medical resources and health care professionals for curing illness, or accepting a woman's decision not to pursue the most aggressive treatment. Preexisting tensions and communication patterns will require work when they are aggravated by a woman's increased dependence. Couples who had managed their resentments and conflicts fairly well simply by leading separate, independent lives will meet their difficulties head-on when illness requires cooperation and unpaid giving of assistance and support. When the spouse's or family's burdens become great or when the illness does not involve pain or visible change, accusations of malingering or using the illness may emerge. Families must grieve for losses of future plans or expected conjoint activities. A counselor will play an important role by helping family members express anger and grief in ways that do not further injure the already-overwhelmed ill woman.

One dynamic that should be anticipated is many women's desire to continue their important function of peacemaker: to smooth the family waters, to ease her spouse's and children's pain and grief, and continue as keeper of family harmony and efficient functioning. Sometimes, this is reasonable and important to the woman's selfhood, but at other times, when the demands of illness are great, she will not have strength or resources to do this for others. Counselors can help families see and respect the ill person's limits and develop family signals by which the woman can indicate when she herself needs rest and care.

By the time a family comes for help, it may have developed a number of painful patterns of resistance and resentment where care of the ill woman is concerned. Restoring balance in the family, enabling even an immobilized woman to play a contributory role in the household and be respected as herself, will require creativity from family members and the counselor. Yet identifying critical functions that the ill woman can continue to perform that have meaning for all members, whether managing household finances, reading to children and helping them with homework, writing holiday cards and maintaining communication with distant family, or deciding what will be prepared for dinner, can restore her credibility in the household as well as her sense of self. Counselors can give each family member a chance to be heard by the others, to express hurts, fears, and frustrations, and to participate in problem-solving.

Work and Productivity

In U. S. culture, productivity is highly valued. Illness, particularly invisible impairment, is often viewed as surmountable by force of will. However, stories of individuals who have conquered disability and gone on to win races or achieve great feats do a disservice to those who clearly are unable or undesiring of such accomplishment. Disability can be stigmatized subtly or overtly when seen as a product of personal laziness or self-indulgence.

Women who are unable to continue the same level of productivity at work or in the home may be hurt by judgments of others and will judge themselves harshly at times. Counselors can help with reality-testing and grief work for women who are struggling with their limits and help them consider the "identity trade-offs" (Charmaz, 1995) that can be part of successful adaptation to chronic illness. Cognitive-behavioral approaches may be useful in helping women face their distorted views of themselves, make realistic appraisals of their capabilities, and practice self-advocacy in interactions.

Cultural differences will affect women's views of the sick role and their responsibilities to others when ill. In Latino or Asian culture, illness and disability may be accepted more readily than in Euro-American groups, but the importance of family involvement in illness decision making is not always respected by health professionals. Asian or Native American women may view their illnesses as having wider meaning of imbalance within the family or their relationships to the natural world. Faith-based rituals may be an important part of a woman's effort to restore herself to full participation. Counselors must elicit and learn about these meanings and practices in order to provide effective support.

Health Care Needs

Counselors will likely be asked to assist with navigating or negotiating health care as the woman and her family seek treatment. Disillusionment and betrayal are common feelings once ill persons exhaust the capacities of the health care system to cure or relieve suffering. For women with low confidence in themselves and low trust in their providers, resignation may be demonstrated in submissiveness, negativity, and hopelessness (Thorne, 1993).

The counselor's task is to assess whether the current interaction is the best that can be achieved under the circumstances or whether old hurt or resentment are getting in the way of productive use of health care resources. A client's style of interacting with health professionals is probably also her style of interacting with other potential sources of support. Much can be learned by reviewing these interactions in the context of counseling work. Role-playing may be useful to bring out a client's emotional responses or misjudgments or reconstruct a hurtful remark of a well-meaning health professional so it can be processed in counseling.

Counselors in long-term therapeutic relationships with chronically ill women might with appropriate permission make contact with their health care providers and develop lines of communication that strengthen the woman's resources without violating confidentiality. Counselors can learn physicians' and nurses' views on what can be expected over the course of a particular illness and experience first-hand the culture of the agency providing the illness care. Greater insight into the client's perceptions and obstacles will be gained. Last, the intimate connections between emotional and psychological well-being and the ups and downs of physical illness should be explored. Women with MS report that emotional upset or stress worsens their symptoms, and likewise the symptoms can produce feelings of helplessness and hopelessness that blossom into full-blown depression, which then exacerbates feelings of weakness and fatigue. In diabetes, which may have no physical symptoms, women report that emotional state can affect blood sugar. Part of reconciling to and normalizing life with illness is gaining insight into these connections and learning to, as MS patients said, "manage your own feelings, manage your daily life, and negotiate the system" (Hainsworth, 1994, p. 240). Depression is a frequent companion of chronic illness and should be taken seriously as a mental health problem, just as illness symptoms that coexist with depression should be taken seriously and not simply attributed to depressed mood (Klonoff & Landrine, 1997). The consequence of not attending to or enhancing women's control over this emotional-physical link may be worsening illness, substance abuse, or suicidality.

Working with women with chronic illness may well be among the most painful and challenging work for counselors. Eliciting gently and with empathy the meanings of illness, the degree to which a woman has reckoned with its impact, and her efforts toward reconciliation with its unending presence in her daily life will bring counselors into a rich and powerful world in which the smallest gifts of comfort or action gain significance. Counselors who develop skills to identify and bolster women's strength in the face of great pain and isolation will gain in their own abilities to face and make peace with life-altering challenges.

5

Pain, Immobility, and Stigma

Illness Burdens

Women with chronic illness share general trajectories of experience, but the unique difficulties and setbacks they must deal with are related to the types of illness, their social and cultural contexts, their sources of support, and their personal history and outlooks. Illnesses vary in their acuity and chronicity: that is, whether they erupt in acute symptoms and then subside for periods of lesser difficulty or remain relatively constant from day to day. They also vary in their social impacts: the extent to which they are visible or invisible to others, how stigmatizing their impacts if visible, and the degrees to which their particular symptoms and demands permit women to continue a socially and culturally "normal" life (Thorne, 1993).

In this chapter, we examine some of the most burdensome aspects of illness: those that interfere with ease of living in the body (pain), that create obstacles to moving and contributing in the social world (immobility), and that interfere with credibility and respect from others (stigma). Acute illnesses and injuries also often involve the burdens of pain, immobility, and stigma. The impact of these particular obstacles on women's lives extends to many different kinds of situations. The pain of arthritis and other chronic pain will be examined; experiences of immobility, including arthritis, Parkinson's disease, spinal cord injury, and stroke will be described; and stigma as experienced by women with HIV and herpes will be discussed. All these obstacles to normal life can lead to social isolation, which is painful, immobilizing, and stigmatized in its own way.

PAIN AND IMMOBILITY: RELENTLESS COMPANIONS

Chronic Pain: An Illness in Itself

Thirty percent of Americans are estimated to suffer from chronic pain, and due to the immobility it causes, chronic pain is the major cause of disability in the United States. Many chronic pain sufferers have no known physiologic cause for their pain. Some may be accused of malingering, even when no psychological disturbances can be found and there is no concrete evidence for such exaggeration (Lubkin, 1995, p. 145).

Illnesses that can bring on acute and chronic pain include cancer, arthritis, lupus, MS, migraine, gastric ulcers, intestinal problems, gall bladder disease, many kinds of muscular or skeletal inflammation or injury, and poorly understood syndromes, such as vulvodynia, which is an acute pain response to even light touch in the groin or vulvar area. Chronic pelvic pain is disabling for some women. Common treatments for pain include narcotic and nonnarcotic medications, surgery, and manipulation or strengthening of muscles and joints. Other types of noninvasive pain control involve skin stimulation: application of heat or cold, massage, vibration, percussion, or electrical stimulation. Stimulation of body energy at key points of energy flow by acupressure or acupuncture also has been used, as have mental and psychological focusing techniques, distraction, visualization, meditation, prayer, operant conditioning, and behavior modification. Psychotherapy is an important adjunct in a program of pain control (Lubkin, 1995, p. 155).

Physicians have been relatively ineffective in helping persons with chronic pain, perhaps because the focus of most health care is on fixing physiologic problems that would cause pain rather than treating pain itself as a problem. Fear of addiction has led professionals and patients alike to avoid or underuse narcotics, and most nonpharmacologic pain relief techniques are as yet poorly researched in traditional medical science and unfamiliar to many health care providers. The woman with chronic pain may be met with scorn or impatience from health care professionals who feel they are without effective tools to relieve her repeated complaints and requests for help. Thus, chronic pain causes suffering not only in the body but in the spirit, as women are abandoned by helpers and lose their capacities to participate in productive life and relationships.

Rheumatoid arthritis (as distinct from osteoarthritis, when individual joints become painful due to wear and tear of aging) is an autoimmune disease in which tissue in joints becomes inflamed, stiff, and painful. As the tissue becomes scarred and damaged, joints become enlarged and immobile. Thus, both pain and immobility are burdens of women with rheumatoid arthritis. Fatigue, anemia, loss of appetite, insomnia, and malaise can also occur. Women are three times more likely than men to get this disease. Most new cases begin between the ages of 25 and 50 (Gregg et al., 1989, p. 132).

Like some other inflammatory diseases, the illness can have long periods of remission, but about half of cases will get worse over time. There is no cure; medical treatment includes a variety of antinflammatory and pain-relieving medications, nonpharmacologic pain relief approaches as discussed earlier, surgery to remove inflamed or damaged tissue, and physical therapy to maintain as much joint mobility and muscle strength as possible. During acute phases of inflammation, rest is the main treatment.

Arthritis and Disintegration of Self

As with MS, arthritis affects all aspects of a woman's life and sense of self. It requires daily accommodation and management of pain and immobility, limits social activity and productivity, creates stigma due to disability and disfigurement, and brings profound uncertainty as to the future. It challenges family and intimate relationships. Dildy (1992, 1996) found that for individuals with rheumatoid arthritis, the onset was "out of the blue," often beginning with a sudden sensation of burning all over and inability to move (1992, p. 77). The diagnosis brought fear of being a burden on others and giving up independence-- being unable to care for others while instead being cared for.

> I walked around looking at people in wheelchairs. It just totally scared me to death because I thought, "Oh God, I'm not ready to do that." (1992, p. 79)

The diagnosis brought the threat of a shattered self. Sufferers described pain as direct and specific, but suffering was experienced as "all-encompassing mental anguish over loss of hope or control." Suffering if unchecked caused disintegration of self: lost dreams, a restricted future, and withdrawal from people and activities to protect others as well as oneself.

> I'd just almost go into shock it was so painful. . . . There's just no let up. I don't know how to describe pain except that it hurts so badly you just don't feel like you can stand it. (p. 84)

Along with pain came mental anguish: feelings of terror, grief, frustration, despair, and self-pity over overwhelming losses and changes in the self:

> You suffer from self-pity and you suffer from how other people see you. . . .
> So if I were to talk about suffering, I would say it's on two fronts. (p. 86)

Women with fibromyalgia suffered in similar ways, due not only to the pain and exhaustion of their illness but to their deep fears of loss of control over their health and therefore their lives. They depleted all their financial, physical, psychological, and social resources in trying to find out what was wrong with them, leaving them with little to rebuild their lives once diagnosed with this capricious and poorly understood condition (Schaefer, 1995).

When Howell (1994) interviewed women with a variety of chronic pain syndromes, she also found that the women who continued to suffer acutely after more than 10 years were those who felt trapped and passive in the face of their problem:

> I have taken more medication and laid around more. I get awfully frustrated at having to lay around doing nothing. I feel trapped by my body and its pain and the medical profession who make you feel degraded and less than human because you need them. No wonder chronic pain sufferers are either severely depressed and/or suicidal. (p. 101)

By contrast, women who took an active role in caring for themselves and managing their pain holistically reported feeling healthier and more confident, regardless of the severity of their medical condition.

Immobility: Being Locked In

Ill persons can be intermittently, permanently, or progressively immobile. One can be immobile due to loss of muscle strength or control, loss of vision or sensory capacity, or pain. Immobility in itself causes other health problems, including decreased heart strength and capacity, respiratory weakness, loss of muscle mass, slowing of the intestinal system, risk of kidney stones, decreased metabolic rate, skin breakdown, and psychological effects, such as depression (Lubkin, 1995, p. 122-124). Social isolation and loss of income and self-worth are other important consequences of immobility. Fear may emerge as another psychological barrier to functioning.

Activity limitations were a major source of suffering for persons with arthritis.

> I felt I was just locked in this body that was suffering and I couldn't get out.. . . I had been so active, you know . . . my husband would have to dress me, and he'd have to go to the grocery store because I couldn't hardly walk. And I couldn't open the car door, 'cause my hands were so sore. (Dildy, 1992, p. 90)

Parkinson's Disease

Parkinson's disease affects approximately 500,000 people in the United

States. It is a condition in which the extrapyramidal nervous system degenerates, at first causing a shaking tremor when the body is at rest. Eventually, it slows voluntary movements and produces overall muscle weakness. Haberman (1996) found that like arthritis sufferers, individuals with Parkinson's disease were faced not only with the emotional connotations of accepting their diagnosis when they were still active in career and family life but with coming to terms with a changing body. They described their bodies as uncooperative, as no longer responding to their usual unconscious intentions of movement:

> I would put my hand up to wave good-bye and I'd put it up and it wouldn't wave. And that was a peculiar feeling. I could lift it and it wouldn't be automatic--and I'd think wave. Oh yeah, I had to consciously do it. (p. 403)

Even simple movements demanded concentration and attention. Complex tasks could be overwhelmingly tedious and frustrating. Individuals with Parkinson's disease faced decisions about whether to continue to work or drive, balancing their accustomed identity as productive and independent with their concerns about safety and ability to perform at their jobs.

They also discovered the intricacies of asking for and accepting help from others without feeling belittled or disempowered. One woman who lived with her adolescent children described how her role as mother changed with her disability:

> They have to do things for me. So, therefore, they sort of tell me how and when it will get done. And I have to remind them I'm the mother and I decide. (p. 409-410)

Parkinson's disease threatened women's self-images as independent, authoritative, competent participants in their worlds. The worsening tremor, stiffness, and weakness create fear of total incapacity, perhaps most threatening to younger women who feel responsible for providing care and income for children, help for coworkers, cooperation and affection for spouse, and contribution to wider society.

Spinal Cord Injury

Traumatic injury of the spinal cord is one of the most feared types of accidents, rendering its victims paralyzed below the level of spinal injury and often unable to control bowel and bladder functions. Nelson (1990) observed a spinal cord injury rehabilitation unit. She found that in the early weeks of rehabilitation, patients were overwhelmed with the impact of their complete loss of mobility. They had lost control over basic conditions, such as privacy and modesty, as they were unable to move to cover themselves and could not manage bodily functions unaided. They had no control over their possessions, routines, sleep, sexual function, or recreation and could not move in bed, in a room, or in their lives. Early in treatment, staff attempted to buffer newly injured patients from the extent of their losses to give them time to adjust. Gradually, the reality of their incapacities would become clear, as they struggled to learn to use machines and tools for eating, toileting, dressing, and moving in a wheelchair. Like Parkinson's disease sufferers, persons with spinal cord injury faced learning how to accept help while maintaining dignity and a sense of control.

Stroke

The impact of a cerebrovascular accident--brain damage due to a blood clot or loss of blood supply to part of the brain--can range from mild transient loss of mobility to permanent inability to understand or speak, paralysis, or death. Stroke is decreasing in frequency in recent years, and its damage can be reduced with new medications, but it remains the most prevalent neurologic disorder among Americans. It is more common in persons with diabetes and high blood pressure and in those who smoke. Black and Asian individuals have a higher risk of stroke than do European Americans, and age increases the likelihood of stroke. Generally speaking, men are more likely than women to suffer strokes, but as women live longer and carry their other chronic diseases into old age, stroke becomes an important issue for women as well (Gregg et al., 1989, p.79).

In the first month after experiencing stroke, stroke survivors were found to immediately set out to regain as much mobility as possible (Folden, 1994). Their first thoughts were to be able to walk independently, manage independently in the home, and for some, to drive again. They grieved their sudden loss; some reviewed how they had taken good care of themselves and been socially active and competent before the event. Stroke sufferers experienced severe fatigue as a major obstacle to their forward progress. It became important to budget their energy and accept shorter hours of work effort. They also described frustration over their lack of control, loneliness due to social isolation and lack of understanding of their experience, and humiliation due to needing assistance with daily tasks, especially toileting. They feared falling or suffering another stroke, being without help when they needed it, and the unknown. Their early goal was to become mobile again to prevent having to accept permanent loss.

Rebuilding a Life Around Pain and Immobility

Reconstructing Self With Arthritis and Chronic Pain

Persons with arthritis not only had to manage their pain; they had to redesign themselves and their places in the world. There were several components to this reconstruction. Arthritis sufferers described needing to make conscious efforts to change thinking patterns toward a positive outlook.

You only suffer to the point that you allow yourself to suffer. A lot of people suffering with chronic disease, I feel like, is between their ears. Their mind allows them because of their background or their experiences. (Dildy, 1992, p. 98-99)

Persons with arthritis who were able to reconcile with it minimized their personal suffering in comparison to other illnesses and focused on overcoming hopelessness and accepting the changes in their lives, bodies, and identities. Arthritis's interruption of their usual activities became a time for reflection and resetting priorities. They described becoming less materialistic and more philosophical and spiritual. They felt more sensitive to the suffering of others, and they described spiritual growth that in turn served as a source of strength. Faith gave them the understanding that their suffering was not meaningless, that all would be well in the end. Their sense of peace was greater when they saw God as aware of their ordeal and there with them.

Arthritis sufferers learned to identify factors that made their suffering worse, including stress, emotional upset, and physical exertion. They also noted that social encouragement, such as support from a husband, friend or family, reduced their suffering and mitigated the impact of stressors on their pain. They observed certain qualities of helpers that were important in relieving pain. These included empathy; being tuned in to the arthritis sufferer's condition; a positive attitude of cheerfulness, caring, and gentleness; and having knowledge and skills to provide effective comfort measures.

Dildy (1992) interviewed two individuals with arthritis who had not succeeded in reconstructing their lives. They had not overcome hopelessness, reached acceptance of their disability, or activated strategies to manage the illness. They were both elderly, widowed, and retired, with little social contact. They both spoke of wishing to die, feeling resentful, not seeing any purpose in their suffering, and feeling that medicine was doing little to alleviate or cure their disease. Without the input from others to provide social validation and encouragement, practical help, and alternative ways of viewing the problem, and without the personal resourcefulness to reset priorities or find spiritual comfort, they appeared stuck in self-pity and resentment.

In reconciling to other kinds of chronic pain, similar values and strategies were described (Howell, 1994). The women who described themselves as healthiest could identify positive aspects of their experience and took charge of their pain management rather than passively depending on health care providers. They felt most helped by health professionals who were willing to listen to them and work with them:

> I think that I get well a lot faster when I'm valued and when I'm part of my healing. That's one of the things I've learned is that I'm really in charge of my health. (p. 101)

These women set out to establish validating relationships with friends, other pain sufferers, family, and health professionals. They needed others to acknowledge them as valuable persons and their pain as real rather than psychogenic. Professionals who doubted their pain or minimized their needs for pain relief increased their distress, sense of isolation, dependency on the health care system, and hopelessness. Some women believed that alternative approaches to pain control, such as biofeedback, did not take into account the real biophysical nature of the pain, and they did not take advantage of these potentially helpful therapies due to this perceived devaluation.

Women who approached pain relief holistically, using a wide range of general and specific strategies to manage pain, reported feeling less distress than did those who relied on only a few strategies. They cared for their whole selves by focusing on healthy eating and exercise; paying attention to stress and upset; integrating mind, body and spirit through yoga; and using journal techniques to dialogue with and come to accept their bodies. Those who balanced rest and activities based on carefully thought-out priorities and incorporated prayer and meditation into self-care were able to feel strong, healthy, and in control of their chronic pain (Howell, 1994).

Slowing Down for Immobility

Immobility also required major adjustments in habit and attitude for persons with arthritis. Daily life was a physical and mental struggle. Putting on panty hose, once a simple process, was now a nearly impossible feat. One woman described putting hers on at night after a hot bath when her joints were more mobile than they would be the next morning. Another told how every task took longer with arthritis:

> Just dressing, like when I first got this I decided I'd try to put on some panty hose one day and it took me 45 minutes to get those panty hose on. And, I said not any more. . . . It's not worth it, you know. So I started wearing thigh highs and knee highs because I couldn't spend 45 minutes every time getting on panty hose. (Dildy, 1992, p. 133-134)

As the uncertainty of a future with arthritis made anticipating and planning difficult, they learned to orient themselves more toward the present and forego commitments in the future:

> Everything is iffy.. . . So, I don't commit. I don't make any really long range plans and that works better because when you make them and you can't, this is a big disappointment. So we just kind of "play it by ear" is the expression. (p. 139)

Coping with the social isolation of arthritis pain and immobility also required modifications of old patterns. With more distant family and acquaintances, withdrawal was a way to avoid having to expend energy to act outgoing when in pain and prevented others from forming negative opinions of them as irritable or depressed when they did not feel well. Or it could be a means of sparing others worry and concern. By contrast, women found great relief and support from being with certain significant others with whom they felt less pressure to be sociable and more understanding and comfort. When validating relationships could be developed and nurtured, they sustained women through the most painful and disheartening times.

The Slow Reintegration After Spinal Cord Injury

Nelson (1990), who studied paralyzed individuals, defined the components of reintegration as transcending limitations and discouragement, toughening against criticism and stigma, and launching into the able-bodied world to make decisions and take action on one's own. This reintegration process was carefully facilitated by the staff at the rehabilitation unit she observed, which functioned as a community with its own social ethos and mores. The process of reintegration facilitated by staff demonstrated the devastating impact of total immobility and the gargantuan efforts needed to overcome it.

In the early weeks, dependency on others was expected and was handled with discretion and respect. Staff assisted the patients to build up their psychological and physical strengths. They began to encourage independence while not allowing frustration to overwhelm the new patient. Friendships were developed. The next phase was helping the patient to transcend the culturally imposed limitations and stereotypes of the disabled. Immobility and all its implications became more and more apparent to the patient as family and friends visited and expressed their dismay and pity. They learned that people in wheelchairs are often treated as invisible, retarded, or deaf and mute. Staff and experienced patients focused on restoring the injured person's sense of self and inner strength. Negative attitudes and hopelessness were squelched, and optimism and pride were fostered. Patients began to be their own advocates and to speak out against those who treated them as disempowered (Nelson, 1990).

Before they could be launched into the world, persons with spinal cord injuries had to be "toughened up" to withstand the stigma awaiting them and to refuse dependency. Staff had learned that unless patients were socialized to resist any unneeded help, they could quickly become an impossible burden on friends and family. Patients were taught to compensate for their physical limitations, become more and more independent both in activity and in decision making, and build strong and mutual relationships that could withstand the strain of their struggle with immobility. For patients who were ready for it, coaxing, teasing, and even criticism were used to introduce the realities they would face.

"Launching" was the final phase in which persons with spinal cord injury were helped to move out into the world outside the rehabilitation center. They began to take their meals in the dining room, to take over more and more of the tasks of their care, and to spend more and more time away from the center with family or others. Progress was measured in achievement of important tasks: transferring in and out of a wheelchair, doing one's own bowel care and urinary catheterization, feeding and dressing oneself, and navigating indoors and outdoors in a wheelchair. Patient autonomy in all aspects of rehabilitation was fostered, with the realization that this would be the key to continued progress after discharge (Nelson, 1990).

Not all illness care builds autonomy so effectively. Persons with Parkinson's disease rarely felt that health professionals were open to hearing about their own innovations and adjustments in managing medications and so forth. They wished that they could share these findings with their doctors. On their own, they developed a tolerance for the unpredictability of the illness and learned to solicit support to accomplish tasks and household chores that gave them a sense of self-worth. The best kind of support, they reported, was when helpers allowed and encouraged them to do things at their own pace rather than intervening and doing it for them, even if the Parkinson's disease made tasks take longer (Haberman, 1996).

Ensuring Forward Progress After Stroke

In the first weeks of recovery from stroke, patients focused intently on achieving progress toward their goal of regaining mobility as the key to self-worth (Folden, 1994). They had accepted the reality of their medical diagnosis, yet regaining function was their goal. Some patients questioned the value of therapies that did not seem to help and wished for more of the interventions that gave them the greatest sense of progress. Increasing control over their recovery was an important way of ensuring forward progress. When a therapist's prediction or goal of limited recovery was less than satisfactory to an individual, he or she would seek to prove the professionals wrong by exceeding expectations. Maintaining hope was essential in the face of the extremely slow progress experienced by many patients. They set goals for themselves and persevered. Although discouraged, one said,

> I am not a quitter--never was. We will stay here until I can get up stairs and then, if I am better, we will go home and see the grandkids. (p. 83)

During this first month of rehabilitation from stroke, individuals were not ready to accept their changed bodies and take stock of their losses until they knew how much they could regain. Over time, the limits of their mobility would become more certain, and the process of reckoning and reconciling would begin.

STIGMA: THE DISCREDITED SELF

Goffman (1993) described stigma as spoiled social identity: the loss of credibility, respect, and value in a social context due to violation of social expectations for acceptable appearance, status, or behavior. Because expectations vary among groups and cultures, stigma can be socially constructed by each group in a somewhat different way. Regardless of the qualities a group defines as discreditable, stigma leads to loss of self-esteem, social isolation, and altered relationships and role performance (Lubkin, 1995, p. 115).

Chronic illnesses often bring stigma along with their many other burdens, because in many Western societies, illness is often seen as the fault of (or a character weakness in) the individual. Even when illness or injury is clearly a bolt out of the blue, recovery is the burden of the patient. The root of stigmatization is the assumption that the different person has not fulfilled her social obligations of self-control and concern for others. Irresponsible sexual behavior and drug use are cause for social rejection because they are associated with selfishness and neglect of one's social obligations of marital fidelity and work productivity. When contagion is also present, stigmatization is even greater. Sexually transmitted diseases, pregnancy outside marriage, and illnesses and infections related to alcohol abuse or illicit drug use are seen as voluntary violations of social codes, and their negative health consequences can be considered fair punishment for these violations.

Perhaps the most stigmatizing health condition in the United States is HIV and AIDS, because it is infectious and seen as the result of irresponsible and illicit sex, drug use, or both. Less deadly sexually transmitted diseases, such as herpes, also carry ongoing stigma. Women with HIV and herpes are subjected not only to the fear, pain, and treatment demands of their illnesses but exclusion from intimate contact or even work or school roles for fear of infection. Feared or actual social rejection leads to self-doubt, isolation, and often to neglect of illness demands.

Herpes and the Dilemma of Disclosure

Genital herpes simplex virus affects an estimated 25 million mainly young persons in the United States (Swanson & Chenitz, 1993). Symptoms often begin with a severe initial outbreak in which many blisterlike lesions appear on and around the genital area, making walking, sitting, urination, and wearing underwear extremely painful. The blisters become weeping ulcers that take a week or more to heal. After the initial outbreak, many herpes sufferers experience several smaller secondary outbreaks a year, often when under stress or ill. The condition is not usually permanently damaging but is highly contagious and sometimes is transmitted even when no lesions are seen.

Because genital herpes is not visible to those other than intimate sexual partners and is not visible at all between outbreaks, women with herpes face the dilemma of how or whether to disclose their condition to actual or potential sexual partners. Disclosure brings the risk of rejection, as well as assumptions of past promiscuity and perhaps lack of cleanliness, and creates the need to decide whether to abstain from sex or use condoms to prevent transmission. Nondisclosure can bring risk of infection of the partner, later discovery and rejection, and feelings of shame or guilt. Faced with the burden of accepting and disclosing this shameful diagnosis, women can lose self-esteem, withdraw from social contacts, and avoid intimacy.

In interviews with young adults with herpes, Swanson and Chenitz (1993) found the young people's lives were marked by instability and change; they were deciding about careers, pursuing or changing jobs, and forming and ending intimate relationships. Herpes affected only the most intimate or potentially intimate relationships, meaning that persons dealt with it privately, responding to an unspoken moral code of doing no harm to a sexual partner. Social lifestyle in this 1980s study was clustered in three categories: "partygoers" who lived a fast-paced social life involving drug use and unstable sexual relationships, "searchers" who sought monogamy but in the process sometimes engaged in recreational drug use or casual sex, and "marginals," less socially active individuals who contracted herpes in their first sexual encounter or within a long-term intimate relationship. The young adults constructed the meaning of the diagnosis of herpes and the options for responding within their social contexts.

Herpes was considered an extremely threatening diagnosis in the 1980s, and the focus of energy in the period around diagnosis was on protecting oneself (Swanson & Chenitz, 1993). On first finding out they had herpes, young people reacted with feelings of dual stigma, of having a socially unacceptable disease and of being labeled as a bad person. Distress was greatest when individuals felt angry and betrayed by the person who infected them, had a frustrating delay in diagnosis, were surprised by the diagnosis, were without a supportive partner, or perceived a negative attitude from the health professionals who diagnosed them. Those with prior experience with chronic illness, who had suspected they had herpes before diagnosis, who had supportive partners, or who perceived a positive attitude on the part of the health professional were less distressed. The health care provider's response had an important impact on the individual's own adjustment to the diagnosis (Swanson & Chenitz, 1993).

After being diagnosed, these individuals sought explanations, examining their relationships and themselves:

> I felt like I was the only person in the world and just felt like totally abandoned and more awful because I had gotten it while I was in a relationship and had been in it for about 5 years and he had lied to me. (p. 281)

> First I was angry at the person who gave it to me, and then I was angry at myself. (p. 281)

The young people then spent a period of time resisting the loss brought on by herpes. As young, mainly healthy individuals at their peaks of social and physical desirability, herpes was often their first enduring physical flaw. They either minimized the impact of herpes, considering it a trivial annoyance, or braced themselves for a very different future in which goals of interpersonal trust, intimacy, and childbearing were now in doubt:

> Now I tend to be real secretive about it. . . . I used to think that people could be trusted, and now it has made me real skeptical about a lot of things. (Swanson & Chenitz, 1993, p. 282)

In interviews with people who had herpes or HIV, Limandri (1989) found that a stigmatizing diagnosis could bring on a period of "free fall" in which loss of the prior known self led to feeling disoriented, acting rashly out of character, or trying to salvage the lost identity. The survivors were then faced with the task of reassembling themselves, or as Swanson and Chenitz (1993) termed it, "renewing oneself." Herpes sufferers began to seek information about the illness, locate and identify with others with the illness, and develop ways of managing the dual risks of rejection or infection within intimate relationships.

To disclose the disease meant owning it as part of the self, reckoning with it. By disclosing herpes, some sought to test their partners' desire for them, to determine whether the partners were interested in them as individuals or only wanted sex. Sometimes, the herpes sufferer initiated disclosure to protect the partner from harm, but occasionally, one was confronted by the partner and forced to disclose, when the explanation of recurring sores or avoidance behavior was inadequate. Some individuals succeeded in not disclosing their herpes, by using excuses to avoid sex during outbreaks.

Gradually, as they found ways to reconcile their identities and their activities to the ongoing fact of the virus, herpes sufferers began to balance their lives by managing symptoms in social, work, and intimate contexts, changing their lifestyles to reduce stress or improve health, and refocusing on aspects of their identities other than as persons with herpes. But when they were rejected by others and did not find acceptance or support, isolation and loss of self persisted (Swanson & Chenitz, 1993).

Who were the risk takers who did not disclose their infection yet continued their sexual relationships? Those who routinely revealed their herpes to potential partners, about a third of the young people in Swanson and Chenitz's (1993) study, had been received with support in early disclosures, had reconciled themselves to the diagnosis, and held positive attitudes toward themselves and their futures. Those who merely accommodated to the disease, another third of the participants, sought to protect their partners but not to discredit themselves unless it became necessary. They only disclosed in an ongoing relationship and only when an outbreak occurred, and they did not have casual or unprotected sex during outbreaks. They were more likely than routine disclosers to feel unfortunate in having the illness and to feel they had little control over its impact. The remaining third avoided disclosure whenever possible and put a great deal of energy into hiding the condition or avoiding interactions and social settings when it could be discovered. They viewed herpes as a permanent flaw with persistent negative impact on their lives. Given that assessment, they either denied themselves social relationships or risked transmission to their partners because they were unwilling to reveal their condition at any cost.

Limandri (1989) found that disclosure was like a swinging gate, which was open, partly closed, or shut tight at different times, depending on past experience as well as present context and perceived receptiveness of the listener. In supportive contexts, disclosure could be sudden or explosive, "venting" in an effort to unload the emotional burden or protect others. Sometimes, this behavior could become incessant or compulsive, perhaps in an effort to garner support. Some individuals dropped hints in hopes of being asked about the stigmatizing condition rather than having to bring it up. When listeners responded with a disclosure in return, future disclosures were made much easier, as the ill person felt that others shared their experience. Nondisclosers had usually attempted it to a minimal degree in the past and experienced negative consequences. They were reluctant to try again for fear of even greater harm, such as loss of a job or important relationship or loss of control over the information. They were still suffering from their losses and sought to avoid even greater pain.

Limandri (1989) also noted that health professionals' responses at diagnosis were extremely important to their patients' acceptance of the illness and later disclosure. Negative responses were rude, abandoning or rejecting, or conveyed inaccurate information. Because health professionals were in positions of authority and were assumed to have knowledge of the severity of the condition, its prognosis, and its impact on one's life, their reactions were taken very seriously and to a great degree defined expectations of others' future reception of the illness.

HIV and AIDS

AIDS was recently the fourth leading cause of death for U.S. women ages 25 to 44 (Centers for Disease Control and Prevention, 1994) and the leading killer of African American women in this age group (CDC, 1995). HIV infection is still considered fatal, but early and consistent treatment can alleviate symptoms and prolong life. Access to and participation in health care become critically important to the survival and quality of life of women with HIV. Poverty, stigma of drug use and the infection itself, and racial discrimination all work against women's access to and comfort with this care.

Being diagnosed with HIV is like receiving dual criminal sentences: of early death and of social ostracism for the life that remains. Langner (1995) interviewed women with HIV who attended support groups. Their initial responses were of terror of dying and yet wanting to die now to avoid the pain of living with the illness: "I couldn't stop crying. I was scared to death. I knew I would be dead soon, and at the same time I wanted to kill myself" (p. 143). As with herpes, some women were completely surprised by the diagnosis of HIV or AIDS, and others had suspected they had the infection, either because of high-risk behaviors or because their lovers were diagnosed. Even when they were certain of their condition, it was difficult to face and accept:

I think I was just blocking it out of my mind--I didn't want to go to be tested. No! I didn't want to face it. . . . I got three kids to raise. I mean, I been married to this man for 17 years. I never cheated on him, and I wind up with . . . HIV? (p. 148)

Once diagnosed, some women launched on a frenzied spree of self-destruction, using drugs and having casual sexual encounters, hoping to escape the pain of the knowledge or maybe die from an overdose. Some were careless about infecting others, thinking that someone had been careless in infecting them.

One mother recalled, "I wanted to die, but I knew I couldn't . . . because of my kids" (Langner, 1995, p. 143). Their children brought mothers their greatest grief, and at the same time they provided a powerful motivation to fight the illness, optimize health, and protect their children from loss. Women grieved loss of the expected rewards of mothering, including seeing children grow up and become self-sufficient, and they suffered with doubt and worry about how to tell their children about their illness. They also worried that if they told their children, the news would spread outside the family. Women pondered when and how to tell them, and simultaneously how to prepare them for a future without a mother. They began to make arrangements for care of the children after their death, and some struggled to improve the quality of their present mothering by giving up drugs.

Reckoning With AIDS

As in other illness and stigmatizing conditions, but in this case facing the shock of "living with dying" (Wilson, Hutchinson, & Holzemer, 1997), the women asked, "why me?" They sought to make sense out of what had happened. Those who had not used drugs or been promiscuous were stunned, but those who had taken risks were also angry, because others had taken worse risks and not become infected. They struggled with the ideas that God was punishing them, yet they reminded themselves that newborns and others who were blameless also got the infection. Women felt isolated and stigmatized even when they had no outward signs of the illness. Some had poor understandings of how HIV could be spread, and all assumed most other people believed it could be spread on contact:

> You can't share with the people out there in the world. They'll mark you. Out there in the world, they don't understand. "Oh my God! She's got that disease! If I touch her, I'll die" (Langner, 1995, p. 154)

Thus, isolation was a primary feature of discovering one had HIV. For some, past behavior, such as drug use, had already alienated them from their families. For others, HIV meant disclosing not only the infection but some other unacceptable aspect of their lifestyles or that of their sexual partners. In addition, some were rejected by the health care providers who gave them the diagnosis and told to seek treatment elsewhere.

Stigma and Barriers to Obtaining Help

In focus group discussions, ethnically diverse women with HIV discussed their barriers to obtaining social services (Seals et al., 1995). The women described fear of negative consequences of even applying for services and difficulty keeping services and obtaining the help they sought. Many had difficulty determining their eligibility for services and finding out how to apply. Some feared using the services due to worry about stigmatization by service providers, exposure of their status to employers or others, and fear of the kind of people who used such services. They described inconvenience, humiliation, and inadequacy in the care that was provided. Services frequently were cut off due to bureaucratic snafus or red tape, and some women went without medical care. Thus, lack of cultural or economic resources not only leaves women without the wherewithal to care for themselves but sets them against dehumanizing and complicated social systems in their search for aid.

Reconciling With HIV

Gloerson et al. (1993) interviewed 15 men and one woman with AIDS who saw themselves as "doing well" with the disease. The first step toward doing well was accepting the illness, which included accepting the fact of the disease and death as a possible outcome and its demands on daily life, knowing oneself, being honest with the self and others that AIDS was a part of one's identity, and reevaluating life priorities. Being physically active in work and with others, being positive in one's outlook, finding a sense of mastery, maintaining a relationship of mind and body through self-healing techniques, taking active steps to participate in one's own health care, and obtaining support from oneself and others were all elements of doing well.

Wilson et al. (1997) also found that after recasting their life goals to take AIDS into account, persons with advanced AIDS could maintain a sense of quality of life even while dying, when they adjusted their hope levels and focused on making their lives and impending deaths the way they wanted them to be. Stigma was a concern early in illness, but as time went on toward death, personal quality of life became more important. They made the most of each moment while at the same time planning for their demise. Time was coveted as a precious commodity as they calculated the increasing nearness of death. Dignity was important in how they looked and conducted themselves even in the last stages of illness. Resolving spiritual issues to gain a sense of connection with community, all of life, or God helped these persons optimize the quality of their living with dying.

On reflection, gay men, the majority of AIDS sufferers who described themselves as doing well, may have the most advantages, if they come from tight-knit, educated, financially secure, activist communities. In this context, the illness brings one closer to the community rather than creating isolation and stigma. For women, on the other hand, especially women in poverty with the responsibility of raising children, the stigma of having contracted HIV from casual or commercial sex or from drug use creates a barrier to accepting the illness and accepting oneself as worthy of care. Lacking the tools of education, cultural majority status, and financial power, women with HIV are isolated from support and potential for growth.

Finding Connections and Support

In reckoning with their diagnosis of HIV and working toward reconciling it with their selfhood and their lives, a support group could be a godsend, giving women a sense of self-worth and healing:

> It's what saved me. It's like pullin' yourself up from a deep dark hole and cleanin' it. It's like my whole inner thing is clean. (Langner, 1995, p. 157)

> I come here . . . and everybody in this room is just like me. And that makes me feel good. I'm not saying that it's good that we have this disease, but good in that I can share with these people. You can't share with the people out there in the world. (p. 157)

The women shared their symptoms and experiences and helped each other find ways to cope with the illness and its burdens. They also became close to women who died, making their own mortality more real. Likewise, Wilson et al. (1997) found that in advanced AIDS, the "presencing" or "showing up" of significant sources of social connection and support were essential for sustaining quality of life as illness worsened.

Mothers with AIDS spoke of how they focused on the present, taking nothing for granted and appreciating time in a new way. Some took steps to achieve goals they had long put off, such as learning to drive or giving up drug use. They became attuned to their bodies and interpreted symptoms and subtle shifts in how they were feeling. Relationships changed, for some by dramatically changing their social networks and for others by enriching and deepening already strong supports. Women who turned their lives around, giving up drugs and prostitution and tapping hidden strengths, discovered entire new selves and embarked for the first time on relationships that were deep and based on equity and honesty. Women living alone faced the dilemma of needing intimacy yet dreading the risk of spreading the infection (Langner, 1995).

Women with HIV have normal needs and desires and participate in interactions, mothering, and relationships, yet their lives are shadowed by uncertainty and death. Langner's interviewees described having continual ups and downs, physically, emotionally, and spiritually, yet continuing to do everyday tasks, pay bills, care for children, give to friends, and organize their affairs for the future (1995, p. 175). At the same time, their weaknesses, medications, health care appointments, and decline over time were constant reminders of their HIV.

For women on the fringes of social acceptance and economic survival, opening oneself to personal growth is not always an option. Stevens (1996) interviewed low-income women with HIV in a west coast city, more than half of whom were women of color. The majority had children, and more than half had not finished high school. These women's completely negative experience of HIV reflected their disfranchisement in many arenas. In lives already overwhelmed by poverty and powerlessness, these women were terrified that HIV would take away their remaining vestiges of self-respect and determination. Their approach was to refuse to let HIV and its treatment take control:

> I refuse to give into the illness. I just do what I have to do. I got a son to take care of. I got a life. I can't be doing all this stuff for the HIV. I don't want it to take hold of me. (p. 147)

To manage from day to day in their difficult lives, these women had to deny the power of HIV, by ignoring or struggling against its symptoms, by refusing to succumb to the regimens recommended by health care providers that would sap what little energy they had for other aspects of living, and by steadfastly focusing on subsistence and their other pressing responsibilities. Health care providers were seen to offer little comfort or information of value while expecting women to submit to time-consuming and embarrassing treatments. Nonetheless, women were frightened and dismayed by their increasing debility and their powerlessness against HIV. Fatigue and wasting, along with other effects of the illness, changed who they were to themselves, and they felt isolated and stuck in futile efforts to fight the progress of the illness.

TEMPERING THE DEMANDS OF CHRONIC ILLNESS

Obstacles to Reconciling With Illness

Pain, immobility, and stigma threaten to prevent women with chronic illness from living self-directed and valued lives and can push even strong and self-sufficient women toward self-doubt, discouragement, depression, and isolation. Given the opportunity, counselors can support women as they come to know the nature of these obstacles and develop strengths and strategies to deal with them. Sadly, some women with chronic pain may be in distress for many years before coming for counseling help. American, society with its faith in science and medicine, leads many women to believe that their pain is caused by a malfunctioning body part that should be reparable by physicians and medical treatments. Immobility, when not perceived as curable, can be hidden or stigmatized as a woman's own fault, making it something private that women do not see as amenable to counseling support. HIV infection can be so devastating in its impact, especially for women with few personal or social resources, that professional help seems threatening, out of reach, or irrelevant.

Naming the Fear and Confronting the Anger

The main foci of counseling will be to whittle these burdens down to a manageable size and identify and build inner and outer resources with which to manage them.[1] Ultimate control or victory may not be a realistic goal here, but instead, the focus of support may be simply to help women feel capable of coexisting with pain, immobility, or stigma while preserving some essential aspects of self. In the process of discussing and naming the feared consequences of their illnesses, women will begin to gain a sense of mastery over their responses and begin to wrestle with the meaning of their suffering. Anger and self-pity are pervasive responses. "Why me?" will be a question each woman will need to face, and their conclusions will vary greatly.

Feelings can shift from day to day. It will be helpful to explore previous experiences to discover the origins of a woman's beliefs about her present illness and the options for management. "Has anything like this ever happened to you before?" is a simple question to open this discussion. Whether the answer is yes or no, personal history will be the key to the meanings women ascribe to the illness. Probing for historical meanings and facilitating ventilation will be early foci of counseling sessions.

Affirming Relationships

To work with women suffering from these extremely isolating and onerous conditions, counselors will need to establish the kind of validating relationships cited by women with chronic pain as a key to their sense of control and well-being (Howell, 1994). As in any counseling work, the relationship becomes a workshop for reintegrating a sense of self and developing tools for other interactions. This is extremely important for women struggling with pain, immobility, and stigma. They need to be believed above all else, to have their suffering recognized and even shared. Once the counselor is seen to really grasp the extent of the woman's physical and psychic anguish and to have appreciation for the sufferer along with strength to move forward with her, work can begin on shoring up self-worth and finding the limits of suffering. To this end, ventilation of grief, anger, and self-pity is a main purpose of therapy for some women: just to have a place where they are valued, the truth of their suffering is recognized, and the listener is not frightened or burdened by the unrelenting pain.

---

[1] For an excellent resource on counseling persons who are adjusting to disabilities, see Marshak and Seligman (1993).

Finding the Limits of the Problem

Forward progress will be founded on reconnection with the strengths and gifts that remain despite the demands of illness. As discussion of the ramifications of living with pain, immobility, and stigma proceed, women can be helped to identify and restructure clearly irrational or overly negative responses. This work can occur only after mutual understanding of the reality of the suffering has been established; otherwise, identifying an overly negative response will be perceived as disbelief. Over time, women can be helped to identify moments of less pain and greater strength. They also can begin to explore situations, social or physical, that increase or lessen their difficulties.

New Connections

Unlocking the prison of aloneness is another major focus of counseling. Women begin this process by sharing with the counselor and feeling understood. The next steps are finding other validating relationships, whether with health care professionals, intimate partners and family, support groups, or special friends. Roleplaying scenarios of disclosing illnesses, and asking for appropriate help or refusing unneeded help, can build a woman's confidence in herself and begin to unlock her social isolation. Clearly, there will be false starts and mistakes, and some newfound social connections may prove to be burdensome or demeaning. Over time, however, these encounters help women to reconnect with the essential, enduring, non-illness-focused parts of themselves and actively seek out persons who strengthen these resources.

Building such relationships requires more than disclosure of the illness. Strength and mutuality in exchanges will be needed if the woman is to avoid self-pity, being perceived as overly needy, or producing burnout in others. As in the treatment of persons with spinal cord injury (Nelson, 1990), "toughening up" is an important preparation for forging new bonds. Counselors can help women determine their own limits and real needs for assistance and work on alternative ways of finding the validation and comfort sometimes sought in accepting unneeded help.

Managing Symptoms and Owning the Solution

The key to reconciling to the burdens of illness seems to be taking an active role in symptom management. Experience and patience will enable women to learn to read their changing bodies and anticipate and manage symptoms. As arthritis sufferers found that physical exertion and emotional stress worsened their pain and immobility, they learned to maintain greater equanimity and moderate their physical activity (Dildy, 1996). Herpes sufferers likewise learned that stress, minor illnesses, and menstrual cycle changes increased the frequency of outbreaks, and they began to focus on better eating habits, overall health, and stress management.

The main obstacle to this proactive self-care may be a persisting belief that someone or something else should be doing this work--that medical innovations or therapies are the only real hope, that the person who gave them HIV or herpes should be the one who pays the price, or that because fate or God determines the course of illness, one's own efforts are inconsequential. Over time, some of these beliefs may loosen, but meanwhile, the focus of counseling can be on reinforcing that the woman is the real expert on her condition and that her efforts are needed as "what we can do in the meantime" or "getting in the best possible condition for God to do His work." In Western cultures, individual agency and responsibility is a pervasive value. A woman usually feels better when she feels some sense of strength and control over her day or her destiny. This may have to be determined experientially, so the counselor may have to set up experiments or contracts to persuade a discouraged, disempowered woman to try an act of self-determination or self-care.

Re-visioning Normal

The eventual target of work with a chronically ill woman is helping her see and achieve a new kind of normal life, one that includes many of the simple rewards of living in the world, sharing with people, and tapping into her own strength and growth. These goals may be accomplished within a wheelchair, in moments of respite from intense work to manage pain, or within the last months of life. Providing ongoing respect, realistic optimism, and opportunities for reflection, grief, and celebration of small victories will aid chronically ill women in sustaining themselves through their trials.

Certainly, there will be phases in chronic illness when clinical depression is apparent, and medication should be considered along with supportive therapy and cognitive work. The grief of coming to terms with a conditions like HIV can lead quickly to suicidality, especially when a woman is without a compelling reason (such as children) to live through the downward course of the disease. To provide effective support, counselors will need to work through their own feelings and positions on euthanasia, assisted suicide, the importance of sobriety for the terminally ill, and so forth. Ethical conflicts may arise in which the client's need for self-determination will need to be weighed against the counselor's need for nonmaleficence. As counselors make the journey with women through pain, immobility, and stigma, personal self-examination, challenge, and growth may be the therapist's secondary gains.

6

Family Violence

Recovering From Trauma Past and Present

THE CONFUSION OF PAIN AND LOVE

A woman who endures childhood abuse or neglect from the family that is her source of self-understanding is denied the opportunity to develop a coherent sense of the world and of human relationships. Women whose intimate relationships in adulthood become violent likewise find themselves in an incoherent world in which loved ones convince them they are at fault for simply being themselves. In this chapter, we examine women's experiences of remembering and growing through childhood traumas and of recognizing and pulling away from abusive adult relationships.

Family is the milieu where a child comes to understand herself as a person, and relationships are the arena where she may define important parts of her adult identity and worth. When harm befalls her in these contexts, her selfhood is shaken or maimed and her capacity to trust herself and others is deeply wounded. Counselors are familiar with the aftereffects of such trauma, which include depression, eating disorders, substance abuse, and other mental health and behavioral disturbances. This chapter will provide a view of women's recollections and their journeys toward healing and growth.

CHILDHOOD TRAUMA

Early Wounds: Betrayal of the Sovereign Self

Many types of harm can befall young girls within their families. These include authoritarian, unloving parents; substance-abusing parents; parents who are violent toward each other; parents who are violent toward children; and parents who have sex with their children. Unfortunately, these sad circumstances do overlap, and some young girls experience all of them. Each has its particular damage, but all result in women's difficulty in knowing, respecting, and relating to themselves.

Alcoholic Parents

In a Canadian study of women whose fathers had abused alcohol during their childhoods (Anderson, 1993), several family patterns were identified. Eight of the 14 fathers were recalled as predominantly "happy drunks," not prone to angry outburst or violence, 5 were predominantly angry when drunk or had a combination of behaviors, 3 were abusive to their wives when drunk, and 1 was physically and sexually abusive to the daughter. Abuse of other family members, especially their mothers, had considerable impact on young girls even if they were not physically abused.

Two kinds of dynamics were apparent in families in which the father actively abused alcohol. In some families, standards were frequently changing and rigidly enforced; guidance was ineffective; and enforcement was severe, forceful, and unpredictable.

> The men always had to be in control. . . . And even when he wasn't drinking, he was in control. (It was like) "you do what your father says, or else!" . . . There was lots of rules; everything was rules! "You do this, this and this, and you don't do this or that!" (Anderson, 1993, p. 93)

These fathers were angry and abusive when drunk and punished family members regardless of their behavior. Poverty and frequent moves were common. Each family member focused on personal survival and avoiding the father's harm, and the family situation was never discussed, even among the victims.

> Nobody said anything (back to my father)! It was just a real hush; never brought up! . . . I think he got (his status) from everyone in the family fearing him. (Anderson, 1993, p. 93)

Mothers in these families were recalled as passive and did not defend their children against the father's harm. This woman and other family members suffered unpredictable physical and sexual abuse:

> I got slapped lots! I can see a little girl's body flying across the room . . . Sometimes I couldn't run, there was no place to go. [pause] Then bad, very bad. . . . I see walls around me. If I couldn't physically get away from him,

then it was abuse: physical abuse and sexual abuse . . . I had a vision of being dragged [to the bedroom]. (Anderson, 1993, p. 95)

Mothers were not available for protection, comfort, or validation of the wrongs suffered by the daughters because they were either withdrawn or suffering themselves.

In other families, members aligned themselves together against the father, keeping secrets from him, and also aligned themselves as a unit against outsiders, orchestrating their public image to avoid shame. The fathers were either angry, happy, or unpredictable as drunks, but none was effective at managing family problems or consistently supportive in responding to members. These families had rigid standards. Expressions of emotion were discouraged, and deceit was common as family members sought to avoid the father's disapproval.

He was sorta like the king, he'd come home and (pause), everybody left. Everybody just sort of ran around trying to please him or whatever and not get in the way. (Anderson, 1993, p. 117)

Young girls in these families were silenced when they felt good about themselves and did not trust their own perceptions of reality or their own worth:

I had gotten this great report card, (pause) and I made the mistake of saying to him I did better on my report card than (name) who happened to be my best friend. . . . And I just got this lecture (from my father) on the fact that I had compared myself to somebody else. . . . And my mom looked at me as if to say: "Why did you say anything?" (p. 120)

This kind of response had lasting effects on the daughter:

Another area I have had major difficulty with is emotions. If I feel any emotions, I feel like I will lose it, I'll go off the deep end; lose control, and won't be able to handle it. (p. 124)

Some of these families were very religious, and daughters learned to seek help from prayer and guidance from the church while adhering to strict social standards. Others learned to simply keep things to themselves and not ask for help and became isolated in their family secrets. Effective social skills were not consistently taught or role-modeled within the household, despite the family focus on social approval.

Anderson (1993) concluded that family functioning was much more influential than the father's drinking by itself, which varied greatly within and between families and produced a variety of behaviors. Daughters linked their adult issues to dynamics within the family, some of which were exacerbated by the father's drinking but most of which involved misuse of authority and deficits in consistency, guidance, and role-modeling. Anderson's conclusion is supported by a recent large study in which the degree or type of victimization experienced by women as young girls was less predictive of harm than was the general emotional health of the family of origin (Draucker, 1997). In contrast, Herman (1992) has claimed that the nature of the traumatic event is most predictive of sequellae, although personality traits and social support, presumably both products of minimally healthy families, are also protective. The common thread predicting survival and healthy development seems to be the degree of strength and connection with which to withstand abuse developed by young girls in their family environments.

When a Father Abuses Family Members

Lombardi (1982) interviewed women who had grown up in homes where their fathers were physically abusive to their mothers. Many of the daughters also had been physically or sexually abused. The majority had grown up in suburban homes with professional fathers; half of their mothers had also been employed. The women recalled great tension and constant argument between their parents. The father's need to dominate the family was a central force. The conflict was exacerbated when the mother was better-educated than the father.

> He pushed her in the corner and took her glasses off and just continued to hit her, punch her in the face. . . . She would always cry and say, "Why are you doing this to me?" but she would never hit him back . . . and she was stronger than him too. . . . I would never understand why she didn't hit him back. (p. 47)

Some had intervened directly as children to try to stop their fathers and had been abused themselves as a result. Many had tried indirect actions, such as distraction, calling for help, helping their mother comply with the fathers' demands, or simply hiding or escaping.

> I kept her from being abused because the dinner was ready when he got home and the house was clean . . . (then) he'd have less to provoke him so I felt responsible if I hadn't done that--if I hadn't made sure everything was OK then I would feel responsible if he hit her. (Lombardi, 1982, p. 49)

The women remembered feeling fear, portrayed in frightening dreams or worrying about their mothers, guilt for causing or not stopping the abuse or for simply existing, embarrassment for the family's problems, frustration when they did not understand the abuse and could not express their feelings about it, and anger at either or both parents.

> When he was beating her I was terrified. I was so afraid that she wasn't going to get up this time you know; this was going to be the time when she was going to be dead. (Lombardi, 1982, p. 52)

As adults, they attributed a variety of effects to having grown up with violence, including low self-esteem, tension, illnesses, difficult relationships with their parents as adults, feeling overly responsible for or close to siblings as a result of their shared trauma, and need for independence from men in their career choices.

> I felt like him attacking her was like he was attacking part of myself. (Lombardi, 1992, p. 59)

> I've never had any self-esteem, not until recently and I always felt like because of the things that he said to me as I was growing up, you know, never a word of praise from him, that I didn't matter, you know, I just wasn't anybody that was important. (p. 60)

Adult relationships were an area of difficulty, as many felt safer and more comfortable with women and mistrustful of men, although some said they had been promiscuous in a search for affection and love. Some had married to escape their families, and all these marriages were short-lived. Some had been in violent relationships that also had ended quickly. All described being hypervigilant and extremely sensitive about violence toward children and adults.

Religious Obedience: Trying Again To Be Good

In a Canadian study of women in religious orders who had suffered recent mental health problems, LaFramboise (1993) found that childhood abuse and neglect had led these women to seek a sense of personal worth in religious life. In therapy, the women had come to see that they had been wounded as children by conflicted, neglectful, or abusive relationships with their parents. They had tried to become good girls who withdrew from conflict and sought to please and serve others. When their search for the ideal self led them to enter the safe and sanctioned structure of religious life, they bypassed the young adult opportunity to find their own voices and threw themselves again into obedience and service.

> Throughout my religious life, I have been striving to earn the love, the approval of those in leadership. I substituted them for my father by being a

good religious, trying to please those in leadership, not making waves or demands. It was the same dynamic as with my dad. (p. 138)

Despite increasing overwork and over-commitment to their duties as teachers, nurses, or chaplains, they felt inadequate and overwhelmed, unfit for their religious vocations. Some felt rage inside but were unable to speak out. In their work settings, they continued to offer healing to others while denying their own suffering, constantly comparing themselves to others who seemed to be calmer and carry out their roles better. They increasingly felt fear, including fear of the dark, fear of being alone, and fear of being punished. Eventually, each reached an impasse when she could no longer function. At middle age or later, they were obliged to withdraw from their duties and seek professional help.

Childhood Sexual Abuse

Undoubtedly, the most tragic and damaging childhood trauma is incest and sexual abuse, often coexisting with other family dysfunctions. To the worst degree, these violations prevent effective self-development. Not being protected, loved, respected or valued, or empowered within their families can result in adult inability to protect their own boundaries, define, respect, or love themselves, or identify or express their own needs. Lack of a coherent family ethic, fear of violence, and their mothers' abdication of their own selfhood further wounds girls and blinds them to their own selfhood.

Cultural and social contexts of sexual abuse. Morrow (1992; Morrow & Smith, 1995) used interviews, journals, art, media analysis, and poetry to study the experiences of a diverse group of women sexually abused as children. She identified cultural norms that continue to promote and perpetuate abuse of girls, all derived from male dominance and female submission. These include social acceptance of men as heroes and rescuers; violence as a legitimate route to effect submission; abuse as supposedly nonexistent in respectable families; women as powerless in families and society; and children as powerless within families, their need for affection making them vulnerable to sexual abuse.

The severity of long-term impact varied among women who had been abused as girls. The harm of abuse could be worsened by religion, which increased women's shame and guilt, and by family loyalty, which prevented them from sharing the secret of abuse. In families where abuse was pervasive, both physical and sexual, and multigenerational, and where alcohol abuse was involved, women suffered the most severe damage. When outside resources of adults who served as comforters or helpers were available, the impact of abuse was lessened somewhat. The younger the age at which abuse began, the greater the mental health disturbances and difficulty reconstructing the past abuse. For some women, rewards for submitting to abuse, such as money, gifts, privileges, and affection, created even more confusion about the harms they had suffered.

Abuse experiences. Women recalled a range of sexual experiences, including sexual talk and exposure of genitals, physical molestation, forced sexual acts, penetration, and other tortures (Morrow, 1992). The abuse ranged from one incident by one person to frequent abuses by a number of persons. The greater the intensity of the abuse and the younger the girl, the less able the women were to remember the experiences or feel any sensation or emotion about them. They recalled extreme pain, sensations of suffocating or choking, and terror. Some recalled feeling pleasure and sexual arousal, which increased their guilt and shame, yet for those who had never been touched any other way than sexually it was comforting at first.

> You know he never, he never whipped me like that again . . . all he had to say was, "Remember how I whip you that time?" . . . Whenever I would resist him at any point, he'd just look at me. (p. 212)

> I was never kissed or touched. So the only touching then was sexual. And that seemed to me like a lifesaving thing. . . . When I was having sex with my father as a little child, it was pleasurable . . . maybe because I hadn't been touched before and needed it--to live. (p. 225)

Abuse caused dreams and memories of terror, mutilation, loss of humanity, and death. Unable to process these feelings as children, women continued to deal with their reemergence. They suffered body memories: physical sensations, such as pelvic pain or stomach pain. Their memories were piecemeal and dissociated, including thoughts, physical sensations, intuition, and emotions. Emotional evidence of abuse was trusted least of all. Some felt their anger and rage would kill them or other people. The women had two major struggles as children and adult women: to keep from being overwhelmed by threatening and dangerous feelings and to manage their feelings of helplessness, powerlessness, and lack of control.

> Being overwhelmed would be like being in a car crash, ripping, screaming metal, screaming people, bodies pierced by shards of hot metal, blood, anguish, ongoing, ongoing anguish. It would be worse than just dying. It would be pain and anguish that goes on, and on, and on, nothing you can ever do would stop it. That's what being overwhelmed by emotions means. (p. 220)

> He stands there. A silhouette at first and then his face and body come into view. . . . He is not always there, but it feels like he might as well be. . . . He seems to be standing there for hours. As if he's saying, you are weak, I am in

control. (p. 222)

Splitting: Shielding the Wounded Self

Bulimia. In four women sexually abused as children who went on to develop
bulimia, Carlton (1992) found that the women continued the childhood pattern of
dissociating emotionally from the physical aspects of their abuse experiences by
developing two adult identities, each serving the other: an experiencing self who
had been abused and was blocked from awareness and a constructed self who went
about daily life.

> As a child, I just floated. . . . It was almost like looking down on somebody
> else, kind of thing. . . . I pretended, well, if I'm not here and I don't feel
> anything, I'm still a good person. . . . That's how I survived it. How could
> you possibly have intercourse with your brother in the afternoon, and then
> sit down for dinner next to him, without flipping out? (p. 101)

Bulimia was a way of dealing with the two selves, in which the injured
experiencing self came out in bingeing, needing food for comfort and self-
nurturing, while the constructed self sought to maintain rigid control over the
outside through maintaining an attractive body image by purging and excessive
exercise, and overachievement in work and sports.

> What I'm realizing is that the bulimia is something I'm using to stop
> feelings. I'm using it to not have to face things. The whole abuse thing, it
> hurts so much to think about, you know. Sometimes I'll have flashbacks of
> the abuse, very, very small, because as soon as I do, I shut them off, I block
> them out. And sometimes I don't even get to that conscious point of
> realizing, without going into a bulimic, you know, into an eating thing.
> (Carlton, 1992, p. 156)

> You have no control over your body when you're being sexually abused, or
> even after you've been sexually abused. . . . And so, you think, the only way
> you can have control over your body is by controlling what you put into
> your body and what your body looks like. (p. 166)

Bulimia was a way of expressing oneself and one's ability to take care of
oneself, yet it prevented growth by creating an overwhelming preoccupation with
food while perpetuating self-hate and a false sense of control. Splitting also
occurred in relationships, in which the woman avoided intimacy by dissociation
and avoiding expression of feelings while continuing to believe in the
importance of being partnered to a male. Revictimization occurred for some
women. Suicidality was another form of self-hate and seeking escape from pain:

Suicide has been my answer for a lot of years, many attempts. . . . I was always just so depressed. Like, I always hated myself. They had all these labels for me, manic depressive and all this stuff. You know, nobody ever got to the problem. It was always just brushed off as something else. Ya, and sexual abuse was the problem. (p. 117)

Body memories during childbirth. The intimate and vulnerable experience of childbirth may bring back responses related to sexual abuse for some women. Parratt (1994) spoke with six British women who had been childhood incest victims and had given birth to one or more children as adults. Three had been unaware of the incest at the time they gave birth. Childbirth provoked memories or responses from their past, as the labor process involved intrusive touching by strangers, vaginal examinations without full consent, pelvic and perineal pain, and denial of privacy. Women described feeling stressed, fearful, sick, and out of touch with the labor and birth process, sometimes without realizing why. Some reacted violently to touch that was meant as supportive, refused to allow procedures such as repair of lacerations to be completed, and pushed the baby away when it was put to the breast. One had a negative reaction to learning her baby was a girl, without realizing why. They found themselves using dissociation to tolerate the birth process, to maintain control and decrease emotions and pain.

It's sort of like, when you're being raped and bashed you've got no control over what's happening and it's the same with giving birth, you can't really control it, the contractions keep coming, you haven't got a choice . . . so like it was better, the only way I could control the pain was by shutting down. (p. 31)

Reckoning With Horror:
Owning Dissociated Experience

Building the Foundation for Change

Herman (1992), in her study of survivors of trauma, noted that not only is terror itself harmful, but the disempowerment and disconnection brought on by childhood abuse must be recognized and remedied if recovery is to occur. She described therapeutic stages of creating safety for survivors as they confront their trauma, facilitating remembrance and mourning, and building reconnection and empowerment. Indeed, all these are seen in women's own stories of recovery.

Constable (1994) interviewed women and men who had been sexually abused as children and who had undergone extensive therapy. Some were initially bothered by fragments of abuse experiences.

I started getting memories. Little flashbacks and body memories and smells. Hearing things in my head that weren't related. Things that people said or noises that were associated with the abuse, but they weren't connected to anything today. I don't know if you know what body memories are like--it's like your body has a memory of its own--and ways that I had been touched that were really abusive, I would start feeling the sensation of being touched when there was nothing there. (p. 70)

Others had a strong desire to change long-standing patterns that were increasingly seen as a source of pain. Some of these individuals were not consciously aware of their abuse when they first sought help. One woman had a weight problem and sensed that something was underlying it. Another had been having troubling dreams and difficulty relating to people; she reported waking up next to her husband and feeling he was a stranger (Constable, 1994, p. 72). All the individuals interviewed by Constable searched for a context to support change, a therapeutic environment that felt safe enough to reveal themselves and explore their pasts. Many had to deal with their families' determined efforts to keep them from exploring their pasts or making changes. Once in a compatible therapy relationship, the individuals spoke of the importance of being accepted regardless of the oddity of their behaviors, which included regression, anger, and resistance. Any interaction that resembled abuse was counterproductive, including being patronized or dominated.

As memories of the abuse began to surface, all the individuals doubted their validity. Therapists accepted these memories and communicated support and encouragement as individuals began to face them, while building the client's sense of control over the memories, increasing a sense of safety. Making connections with other abuse survivors was also helpful to many individuals, whether through groups or reading personal accounts. As they began to break down their lifelong feelings of aloneness, the power of the abuse memories began to shrink.

Before individuals could fully confront and deal with their abuse memories, they had to build internal resources. Participants spoke of needing to increase their self-awareness, including of their feelings and reactions to people and situations. They worked to separate feelings based in the present from reactions of self-protection rooted in the past. Self-observation, writing, and discussion helped toward self-awareness. They also worked on identifying what they needed from others and their environment, and on connecting feelings to needs. Individuals learned to nurture and care for themselves, including how to soothe themselves when in pain, how to take time for themselves, and how to set limits in relationships with others. They also learned how to pace themselves in facing and internalizing the reality of their abuse. For many who had grown up without any sense of deserving attention or nurturing, it was difficult to accept that they deserved self-care.

Reconnecting With Abuse Experiences

Once the abuse survivors began to recover the memories and reassemble them, they found that they were more extensive and more traumatic than previously realized. Some individuals could recall the events but had no awareness of their physical or emotional responses. Some discovered that their abuse had begun at a much younger age than they had previously realized or involved more events or worse trauma. The impact of recovering complete memories, even brief flashes, was devastating.

There was some days that I did not think I could function . . . I would spend [time] just crying and not wanting to see people--this outgoing extrovert who was always on the go--And a lot of hate and anxiety . . . it all sort of bubbled to the surface, and it had to be dealt with. (Constable, 1994, p. 139)

Some individuals had anxiety attacks or physical sensations that terrified them or saw visual images that were disconnected from anything they could recall. Therapists were invaluable in creating frameworks for understanding the memories and sensations that arose over time. It was helpful simply to see that they were experiencing memories of abuse that were fragmented, in a sense, for their own protection.

As they learned to manage their returning memories, individuals felt increased control over the memories and their reactions. Some found that art or dance were safer or more fluid modes of expression of their feelings, especially if they had been threatened in the past not to speak of the abuse. Over time, the memories became less frightening and more interesting and useful, as individuals worked to reassemble their pasts. Therapists were helpful in teaching techniques such as dream work and journaling for capturing and ordering memories and in suggesting interpretations or new views of memories to open new avenues for understanding.

Some participants despaired of ever feeling a connection with their parents again. Their increasing rage and sadness were difficult to deal with.

I've felt more than once like I was drowning. . . . Unless you've been through it, you can't know the intensity of the emotion that's involved and just how devastating it can feel to realize fully the fact that the people who were responsible for you being born are the very ones who hurt you and hurt you so bad. . . . I felt no bond at all. (Constable, 1994, p. 155)

To manage the intensity of emotions, individuals tried to learn to use the support of others in the present. This required reckoning with their present capacities: remaining aware that they were no longer the abused child and could use adult strengths to deal with their suffering. They worked to remember that their present environments were safe and their present selves were capable and powerful. With these realizations, progress could be made toward reconciling with the frightening past. And as they recovered many negative memories, they also found that positive memories returned as well. Individuals felt increasingly reconnected to themselves and gained a sense of increased solidity in their relations with others.

Reconciling With Childhood Harm: Rebuilding a Worthy Self

Constructing a New Way of Life

Draucker (1991) interviewed women who had been incest victims and had made considerable progress toward healing. These women spoke of needing to "construct a personal residence" for themselves, a safe and personally satisfying life, in a process that resembled designing and building a new house. They built a new relationship with the self, not simply viewing themselves differently but treating themselves better, moving from criticism and self-neglect to self-acceptance and caring. They also worked to move attribution of blame for the abuse from themselves to the offenders. They learned to regulate their boundaries, controlling who would be part of their lives, learning to ask for and accept help when needed, bringing in others who met their needs and were positive influences and excluding those whose effects were harmful. They sought to set new parameters in relationships and to maintain a more equitable degree of control. Some moved toward influencing their communities, personally reaching out to other abuse survivors, becoming advocates for children and other less empowered groups, and working to increase public awareness of abuse.

As Constable's (1994) sexual abuse survivors worked toward reconciliation with their abuse, they began to place blame where it belonged--but only after many months and years of hearing from therapists and others that they were not at fault, and after much work to understand who they were and what they had endured. Realizing that they been powerless in the early situations brought back feelings of anger and hurt but corrected their perspective on the abuse. They also worked to clarify the connections between past abuse and present difficulties and to become reconciled to their faults and unhealthy reactions as understandable yet changeable. Once they could acknowledge their mistakes without feeling devastated, they could begin to try new behaviors with the help of therapy. Substance abuse and manipulation of others could be seen as survival behaviors from the past, not personal defects, and thus became subject to change.

Seeing New Possibilities

As their understanding of their families increased, the families lost their role as potential sources of comfort and referred identity, leaving the individuals to strike out on their own to become someone new.

> You have to decide whether the creature of the abuse is going to control your life, or whether you are going to build somebody else in there . . . somebody that you really like. (Constable, 1994, p. 178)

With new sense of the possibility of positive identities, survivors of childhood abuse began in small ways to make changes in their lives, including recovery from substance abuse, improvement in work habits and behaviors, expressing needs and maintaining boundaries in relationships, and managing emotions. Some left what had seemed promising career tracks when they realized they had been doing it based on someone else's understanding of what they needed to do.

As skills increased, Constable (1994) found that ability to handle more intense memories also increased, and as these issues were dealt with, the journey became less fraught with ups and downs and more rooted in the present. No survivor felt that there would be an end to the process; they accepted that their injuries would be with them for the rest of their lives but that they would be able to manage the pain and get on with other areas of focus. Reclaiming oneself was the ongoing task:

> I feel more alive. I feel more human than I ever felt in my life before. I never felt that I was my own person before. . . . For the first time in my life, I realize that I am entitled to my life, and I don't have to live my life for everybody. (p. 214)

INTIMATE PARTNER VIOLENCE

Over 2 million women are battered each year in the United States (Newman, 1993), at least 2 of every 6 women in their lifetimes, and 1 in 4 Canadian women experiences violence at the hands of an intimate partner (Merritt-Gray & Wuest, 1995). These figures are probably grossly underestimated, as underreporting of at least 40% is suspected (Newman, 1993). The prevalence and underreporting of male battering of their female intimate partners can be understood if we consider that this violence, like sexual abuse of girls, is tacitly supported by Western cultural and social systems in many ways.

Many women are raised to believe that they need to be partnered with a man for social respect and personal and financial security. The wife and mother is often given the role of maintainer of family functioning, harmony, and unity.

Loyalty to one's family of origin and one's husband's family is also valued. A woman who is beaten is often blamed for her abuse as having failed at one of these expectations. Because women are viewed as weak, dependent, and incapable in many arenas of society, their feelings of guilt, helplessness, and low self-esteem further perpetuate abusive relationships (Landenberger, 1989; Pilowsky, 1993).

In Latin American cultures, cultural values of *respeto* and subservience of wives to their husbands create even more powerful obstacles to leaving abusive relationships. Taking possession of a wife is an overt part of some marriage customs:

> My mother used to tell me once you choose your man you must remain with him. You must remain and obey whatever he says, he is the responsible one . . . . In Guatemala we used to say that the price of a wife is thirteen cents. . . these are the thirteen cents that the husband pays for us when we get married. . . . They pay for us when they put the ring on the finger. . . . They also put around our bodies a lasso, a metallic lasso. . . . These are customs, I guess. (Pilowsky, 1993, p. 106)

In a Canadian study of Latin American women who had left their abusers, Pilowsky (1993) found that the women had been raised to believe that they an ethical duty to be a good wife, good mother, and to sacrifice their own needs for the family. One related an old Spanish saying, *"El hombre is de la calle, la mujer es del hogar"* (p. 106), meaning that the man belongs in the street and the woman in the home. Violation of these tenets would bring shame and worthlessness, as well as disgrace on one's family of origin. Good mothers gave their children a father, to provide a symbol of familial respect. *Respeto* required deference of children to elders and a wife to her husband, and these behaviors brought *respeto* on the family when judged by outsiders. If a wife left her husband, their children would be deprived of respect. Good women value men-- whether infants or elders--over women of any age. Good women are married, and good wives devote themselves to fulfilling the wishes of the husband and preserving the integrity of the family.

In many communities, belief in family sovereignty and privacy perpetuates neighbors' and family members' silence about even blatant abuse. Ineffective or punitive police responses and unwillingness of health professionals to recognize and intervene in domestic violence are consequences of these beliefs. Lack of social resources to support women who leave abusive homes is another barrier. Social isolation of families due to geographic dislocation or rurality, cultural isolation in diverse neighborhoods, and separation from extended family and friends can perpetuate women's belief in the normalcy of their situations and their ignorance of resources for assistance. Some women may be pressed by their partners to quit their jobs and drop outside friendships, increasing their isolation. Other personal history and social problems can also increase women's vulnerability to immobilization in violent relationships. Although women from abusive families of origin are no more likely to marry abusers than are women not abused in childhood, women from abusive families may be more likely to tolerate prolonged abuse (Landenberger, 1989).

Becoming Immobilized: Entry Into an Abusive Relationship

Women in abusive relationships have described themselves as self-sufficient, competent, and sociable, yet they adhered to the belief that accommodation of partners' needs was important in relationships (Lempert, 1994). Landenberger (1989) found that women were led into these partnerships due to their strong desires for loving relationships. They noted certain warning signals in the early relationships but chose not to pay attention to them. Gradually, they were bound into the relationships and more deeply committed and invested in them. Early in a violent relationship, a woman made concerted efforts to smooth over conflicts and give the partner what he wanted, believing that they truly loved each other and with work they could make things better. Tension began between the woman's need for affection and hopes for a happy relationship and the growing reality of abuse. She searched herself for personal flaws that could explain the violence. Although some at this point began to consider the idea of leaving, they did not think seriously about carrying it out.

Latina women were led by their husbands to believe that they were crazy and fools (Pilowsky, 1993). Believing that their only purpose in life was to nurture a family, fearful of deportation as illegal immigrants, and doubting their own capabilities, they were bound into violent relationships by social and cultural pressures as well as the interpersonal dynamics within the home. Shocked at first that their husband would harm them, they built up layers of denial and minimization when they could see no alternative.

In analysis of a narrative from one abused woman, Lempert (1994) noted that even in her speech patterns, the woman took on a passive and distant stance when discussing abuse. She described an almost involuntary process of social pressure and coincidence that brought her and her husband together and revealed their suitability for each other. She could recall certain warning incidents but not their context because she was blocking out evidence of a problem:

> I was driving in the car with him and he got mad at me and I don't even know why and he made me get out of the car . . . in the slum area and he just left me. (p. 419)

She felt no strength of will and simply bent to his force, wanting to go along with his wishes. More and more, she stifled her anger over his acts of control.

Violence that had been unpredictable became regular. She remained with him for more than 7 years, for many reasons:

> Part of me believed he wouldn't do it again, part of me was so embarrassed... and part of me was scared. I wasn't working now. Now I was gonna have a baby . . . where was I gonna live?. . . I want this baby to have a father and everything, and I guess I just thought, "Well, I can make it right." (p. 428)

These highly practical rationales bind many women into abusive relationships. Their real economic dependence, the needs of their children, and their desires to preserve the positive aspects of the relationship are powerful incentives to keep working to make things better. These motivations are made more powerful as women experience shrinking self-esteem, embarrassment about having made the mistake of getting into the relationship and missing earlier chances to act, and increasing doubts about what was true and what was acceptable.

Living for Others: Surviving Without Self

In a study of rural Canadian women who had left abusive relationships, Merritt-Gray and Wuest (1995) found that women counteracted the reality of their abuse by relinquishing parts of themselves:

> I had taken his ways into me. I molded myself into the situation instead of still keeping my own self. I had let him put me down so far that I was a part of what he was. (p. 403)

The women let go of their self-respect, their independence, and eventually their dream of a stable, happy relationship. They were too embarrassed to acknowledge abuse to family and friends, and they feared humiliation if they confided in anyone in their close-knit rural communities.

Practical and psychological efforts to separate from or minimize abuse enabled women to survive in violent relationships. Psychological strategies ranged from dissociation and denial (Lempert, 1994), in which a woman distanced herself emotionally from the abuse, to efforts to figure out what was wrong with herself and fix it. When they dissociated from abuse, women were able to block it from awareness or memory, although they knew it was wrong. In this way they could endure for years (p. 434).

Over time, women's prior understandings of themselves and the version promoted by their partners became more and more disparate, and the valued self became dormant as women put conscious efforts into meeting their partners' needs and complying with the personas imposed on them by their partners.

Shame at what must be at least partly their fault continued to prevent them from telling anyone about the abuse:

> I know I didn't deserve it but then why was it happening? I mean I must have been contributing somehow. . . . So, I didn't tell anyone. I didn't have any trust and I was ashamed for myself. (Landenberger, 1989, p. 217)

Some women tried to reason with their abusers, explaining how much the violence hurt them, begging them to stop, offering to help them seek therapy (Merritt-Gray & Wuest, 1995). These efforts were based in the belief that the abuser could change and the relationship could then be preserved. In the repeating cycle of escalating tension, violence, and recovery, men who were remorseful and affectionate after episodes of abuse offered enough hope of reform that the woman persisted in the relationship. Some women did fight back against their abusers. This resistance included threatening or carrying out return violence, threatening other harms, separating the abusers from the children, calling police and using legal protections, and being emotionally abusive to their violent partners.

When all her efforts failed to stop the abuse, a woman began to realize that her partner was not going to change and that the partner's message--if she changed, the abuse would stop--was false. Some continued to use numbing strategies, such as drug and alcohol use or dissociation, to endure what they knew was a hopeless situation. Gradually, however, those who eventually broke away began to disengage from their partners' definitions of the situation and to consider reclaiming their selfhood. Women who had been abused in childhood took much longer to arrive at this conclusion, perhaps because they were skilled at dissociating from the abuse or because they had had little experience of entitlement to an independent, acting self.

Latina women faced strong cultural prohibitions against accepting help outside the family when it meant going against the husband's wishes. When other women in their families or cultural groups described tolerating violence, they tried to see it as normal. Yet they too arrived at a critical juncture when they realized that their situations would not change and that despite cultural support for the sanctity of the family, there was also support for the value of women. As one woman said:

> I remember looking at him as if for the first time in 8 years. I told myself if I continue this relationship, I am denying myself. I had this illumination, you can say. (Pilowsky, 1993, p. 103)

Reckoning With a Wrong Situation

To justify breaking free, women had to internalize the belief that they were experiencing domestic violence and that it was wrong. With this understanding, they could begin to connect with other abused women and use available resources. Yet the process of leaving was long. It involved gradual change and often many attempts to leave before women were able to stay away for good (Landenberger, 1989).

Family and friends offered both supportive and negative input (Merritt-Gray & Wuest, 1995). When helpers described the abusive partner as crazy or no good, the woman felt supported in their new definition of the situation, but when the helpers pushed the woman to leave, they increased her feelings of incompetence. Yet communicating with an outsider was an essential step in beginning to pull away. Employers could be especially helpful for those who worked outside the home (Merritt-Gray & Wuest, 1995). When an employer had faith in the woman's work potential, it could serve to build the woman's sense of her skills and capability.

It was a great struggle to overcome their desire to preserve the family for the sake of the children. This was especially true for Latina women, even when they recognized the wrong of abuse.

> I wanted the children to have a home, *una buena familia* . . . *con respeto* (a good family, with respect) . . . even if there were fights, they still had a family . . . the support of a father. (Pilowsky, 1993, p.108)

Often when they approached others from their culture and disclosed the abuse, the Latina women were encouraged to go back and talk to their husbands, to get the priest to talk to him. When these efforts failed, women who eventually broke away felt they had no recourse but to accept that the man would not change. They began to reexamine their value of self-sacrifice for the sake of the marriage and to see that although it was good to give to others, it was not good to endure humiliation. To risk death or insanity or incarceration of either parent was harming the children, not helping them (Pilowsky, 1993, p. 118). Some women became angry, at themselves and their partners, for perpetuating the abuse (Landenberger, 1989). Using confidence built up in positive experiences outside the home, they used their anger to take action.

Ignorance of available resources was an obstacle for many women, particularly for immigrant Latinas who not only had limited exposure to the concept of domestic violence as a social evil but were often unaware of shelters, legal help, or strategies for starting over outside marriage. Their inability to speak English was a barrier and decreased their confidence in their ability to manage on their own. They feared police due to negative experiences in their countries of origin and did not see themselves as entitled to protection by the laws of their new country.

Isolation from outside support, due to cultural differences, control by the abuser, or social conventions of family privacy, was a major obstacle all women had to overcome in seeking help. When they finally found a compassionate friend or professional and began to accept that they had worth and were not alone, the disengaging process began to accelerate. Some women called the police and finally took them up on the option of obtaining a restraining order or accepting a referral to a shelter. Some took the children to stay with a friend or family, despite some hosts' urging to go back and try again. Gradually building experience away from the home, women grew in their confidence and hope even as they grieved for lost comforts, beliefs, and dreams.

For both Anglo and Latina women, reckoning with domestic violence meant giving up an entire structure of belief about women's roles, the refuge of marriage, the definition of good mothering, and one's own ability to soothe and please others and make things right. Women struggled to make the transition between faith in themselves as dependent yet fixers of interpersonal problems and faith in themselves as independent and yet unable to rectify the core of their life, their marriage. Many cycles of believing and disbelieving, hoping and hopelessness, tolerating abuse and being infuriated by it, and leaving and returning were required before women finally were able to leave for good and attempt to rebuild their lives.

Reconciling: Reassembling the Shattered Self

In a transition period between starting to counteract the abuse and never going back, women spent more and more time psychologically and physically away from the home (Merritt-Gray & Wuest, 1995). This enabled them to see what resources were out there for them, how they felt away from their partners, how the children would cope with leaving, and how they would feel about themselves. They began to strengthen and consolidate their understanding of what others may have seen long ago: that the abuse was not their fault, and that there was no hope of change or reconciliation. Finally, they could see that leaving was the best thing for their children as well, either because the children were becoming stressed and troubled in the abusive family (Lempert, 1994) or because they managed well enough with the care of the mother alone.

Yet there were always tensions between staying and leaving. Newman (1993) found that most women in a battered women's shelter planned to return to their abusers. They had left home for the sake of their children, as they had done many times before. They had noticed their children becoming withdrawn or violent and doing poorly in school, and they sought shelter or a safe respite. Most had little money, were unemployed, and had children to support. While in the shelter, they considered their options and concluded that the resources outside the home were inadequate to enable them to leave and rebuild. Furthermore, they felt leaving would endanger their families of origin, if the abuser retaliated. They felt essentially helpless and afraid of the unknown; they blamed themselves for the abuse and held hope that things would improve at home. In their view, the police, health professionals, and social service agencies either ignored their problems or did not have the capability to make a difference.

In contrast, women who had been in a shelter and eventually became independent (Montgomery, 1994) resorted to homelessness in search of a better life for themselves and their children and successfully found support in the shelter. Their journeys were rooted in stubborn pride, stoic determination and clarity of focus, belief in living by moral rules of right and wrong and in being able to survive with very little. In a positive shelter environment, they learned about their own personal strengths, and they developed interpersonal skills and a sense of belonging and contributing to a group: "They sought my input on everything. They thought I was responsible" (p. 41). Some had to go through the motions of generosity and kindness before it felt real. Gradually, women learned how to participate in nonexploitive relationships. They found new appreciation for their relationships with their children.

In the initial years after leaving an abusive relationship, women focused on shelter, food, income, children's health, and overall, their safety (Landenberger, 1989). Many felt a pull between the old life and the new, often bleak situation, and they maintained contact with their partners and made excuses to themselves and others for why they were staying away. Yet, small kernels of self-worth they had grown in the period of breaking free sustained their hope and determination. Both this inner drive and external resources were important to surviving.

Women's skills and determination can be sorely tested in the initial period after leaving. Many abusers become more dangerous as they seek retribution and to reclaim their "property." Battered women's shelters and safe homes can be life-saving, yet shelter living is an uncomfortable and often humiliating experience. Children act out or grieve as they struggle to adjust to new schools and surroundings without familiar possessions and family, women are subject to myriad rules and restrictions, privacy is nonexistent, and pathways to independence seem faint at best. Strength and hope are sorely tested.

Grieving for Many Losses

After leaving an abusive relationship, a woman grieves not only the loss of her relationship or marriage with its good parts and loving moments, but the loss of her home, possessions, community standing, economic security, and ultimately her former identity. She grieves for what her children have endured during the abuse and what they are enduring in new, often deprived circumstances. She also grieves for the beliefs that had sustained her during the abuse--that staying was the right thing to do, that her partner could change, that she could make a difference for him and could make it work, that humans are trustworthy and good, and that her children needed a father in the home.

Building an Independent Self

Over time, Anglo and Latina women worked to revise their understandings of their lives to make sense of the abuse. They struggled to rework their identities, often through profound depression and despair. At the same time, survival forced them to take risks and learn new skills such as interacting with strangers, using the legal system, managing money, keeping a job, learning a new language, and single parenting. Small successes and simply living though many hardships gradually provided women with the evidence that they were capable and intelligent (Montgomery, 1994).

Germain (1994) created a community journal for residents of a shelter for battered women. The entries reveal the extent to which women were starting from scratch to find their new selves:

Time knows no meaning of how long it takes to find peace of mind and forget your mistakes. (p. 207)

I've learned what it means to be and feel human again. (p. 210)

When you come to terms with your own self you are able to reach out to others. (p. 210)

Today I know what Dr. Martin Luther King meant by "Free at last" . . . I feel delivered. I feel born again. Free to be me. . . . Here I found peace and found myself. (p. 210)

CONCLUSIONS: HELPING ABUSE SURVIVORS

Battered women are most likely to leave their abusers when they have economic, legal, and social resources to turn to outside the home (Ulrich, 1993). But to make use of these resources, changes in self-concept are also needed. Counselors can participate in this rebuilding by providing women with the opportunity to be heard and believed and to process through their own decisions.

Gradual awareness of the reality and wrongness of her abuse is part of each woman's recovery story, whether from childhood trauma or domestic violence. Counselors must commit to the long haul of accompanying women on the road to recovery of their pasts and reworking their definitions of what happened.

Short-term counseling interactions, such as those with shelter workers or victim assistance programs in the courts, should be accompanied by opportunities to build trust over the long term and do major work on self-concept and relationship patterns.

Assessing safety and signs of escalating violence is important at the first contact (Stuart & Campbell, 1989). When a woman seeks help in an emergency, she should be helped to go to a safe place (a friend, family, or shelter) directly from the office or agency. Yet this help should be given in the form of concerned suggestions rather than directives, to avoid replicating women's experience of disempowerment and failure. Women living with abusers become adept at recognizing when their partners are becoming more dangerous. Counselors can bolster these perceptions and reiterate their personal concern as well as their faith in women's judgment.

For a woman to leave her abuser, she has to want to leave him and believe she can do it and that there is hope for a better life for herself and her children outside the relationship. These are all areas for counseling work over the long term for women still living with abusers. Women can be brought back repeatedly to their own resourcefulness in attempting to pacify the abuser, their courage and perseverance in surviving the abuse, their ability to give to their partners and their children, and the strength embedded in that.

Over time, women can be helped to learn by experience that they have the capacity to leave. This can begin by discussing options for temporary shelter and making safety plans for emergency escape. Simply taking steps toward development of a plan can reaffirm a woman's capability and resourcefulness. Counselors can suggest places for storing records, keys, money, or other resources to be used if the woman needs to leave the home. At the same time, women can strengthen their senses of self and their potential for independence by seeking education or job training. If this seems impossible because of the controlling action of the abuser, simply examining this barrier may help a woman see how limited her life is within the relationship. Considering what little is left of the relationship is another strategy by which women come to realize that they have little reason to stay (Ulrich, 1993).

Contact with other abused women through hotlines, groups, or visits to shelters can be immeasurably helpful if the woman is willing. Books and films may also strengthen her belief that she is not alone and that women have built new lives after abuse. Positive encounters of all kinds demonstrate to a woman that she is worthy of caring, that she has something to offer, and that there are safe places and safe relationships that can be hers outside the abusive relationship. For some women, pulling away from the abuser is a gradual process of supplanting that relationship with other more positive ones. For others at risk of life-threatening harm, the break must be sudden and is often more traumatic due to the degree of disempowerment the woman has suffered.

Although their trajectories of healing may differ, both women abused in childhood and those abused in adulthood must rebuild their understandings of who they are and how they relate to others. Their power to influence their own future must be tapped, and the impact of victimization on their ongoing behaviors must be examined and addressed. This is a long therapeutic process and requires in-depth understanding of the experiences of abused women, the psychopathology that can result from long-term abuse, and women's common responses as they reclaim their past and recover from it. Counselors are in a position to provide a safe space for women to experience healthy, long-term egalitarian and nurturing relationships.

7

Eating Disorders and Addiction

Changing Deeply Rooted Patterns

SILENCING PAIN: SUFFERING AND SELF-CARE

Women with eating disorders and women addicted to alcohol or drugs share the strategy of using the physical body to silence emotional pain. Many of these women have suffered childhood trauma, as described in the previous chapter. This chapter focuses on some of the possible aftereffects: the difficulties caused when women attempt to care for their hurt selves through eating, avoidance of food, or use of addictive substances. The hurt becomes worse and worse as these efforts cause their own damage. Recovery involves learning to recognize and face honestly the hidden pain and the behaviors it has prompted and finding healthy ways to care for oneself that respond to rather than silence one's feelings and one's voice.

Addiction is a behavioral illness in which social disparities play a large part in recovery. Although women from all social strata become addicted, those who grow up in impoverished, violent, chaotic households revolving around drugs may never have learned basic tools for building a self-sufficient life. Illicit drug use creates an outsider economy, social structure, and lifestyle, little of which is transferable to conventional life. Middle-class addicted women may be deeply scarred by family trauma, but if they have absorbed the basics of an education and have an understanding of how to pursue goals, their economic path out of addiction is a much easier one.

Anorexia and bulimia reflect the lasting damage that can occur even in childhoods of privilege and plenty. Young girls learn that beauty brings great rewards, and being thin creates feelings of worth and desirability that women discover they can control. This message is greatly reinforced by the commercialization of beauty as a commodity that can be obtained through products and behaviors (Hesse-Biber, 1996). Personal and family problems are sidestepped by shifting focus to this other arena: the drive to achieve beauty and approval by overcoming the power of food, often accompanied by a drive to achieve superiority in other areas as well. What you do and how you look become all-important, rather than who you are. Addiction and eating disorders often have very different social contexts and lifestyles, yet they are both destructive efforts to care for the self while blunting its means of expression and growth.

EATING DISORDERS: POWER OVER SADNESS

Suffering in Silence

In studies of women with anorexia or bulimia, childhood abuse, loss and loss of control were found to be common experiences. Kasperkowski (1991) interviewed four white middle-class Canadian women with anorexia or bulimia. One woman had a degree in psychology and worked as a counselor. Her childhood had been fraught with fights between her parents and constant criticism of her. Her family was very focused on appearances. Her mother put her on diets from a young age. By her teens, she was controlling her weight by bingeing and starvation.

> I was lousy at tennis. I didn't have a lot of friends. I didn't have boyfriends. So, I felt like I was really unacceptable and I was pretty unhappy. And I think that I decided that if I was thin, I'd be acceptable . . . I'd be popular. . . When I was young . . . the only way I could get any control, I think, was by sort of taking my own body and saying, "No, I'm not doing this." . . . It's a powerful feeling to feel that the rest of the world needs to eat and you don't . . . That you're kind of impervious to needs, which is very dangerous because you end up feeling that you don't have any needs. (p. 92-93)

All four of these women described being silenced by their families of origin, even forcibly, as when one woman had her mouth taped shut by her mother (Kasperkowski, 1991, p. 101). All described their mothers as controlling, critical, and unable to hear their daughters' needs. Their fathers were distant or abusive and sometimes frighteningly angry, and later relationships with men were difficult as well. Gulley (1991) interviewed U. S. women with anorexia nervosa, who also echoed family issues of abuse, chaos, addictions including work addiction, and parental absenteeism. The mother was the disciplinarian in most instances. The women described having little sense of who they were apart from their mothers' expectations of them.

Diet for Control

Young women in the throes of confusion and self-dislike found dieting a useful solution. It gave them a sense of being able to control themselves, and initial weight loss brought attention and praise from others. Perhaps for the first time, they began to feel they had power: to look good, to be liked, and to be free from the temptation of food and the pain of emotional distress. By not feeding their bodies, they numbed other painful feelings as well. The diet began to take control, and women began to fall into cognitive distortions. They saw fat in a too-thin body; they sought to hide their private obsession.

I feel light and free when my weight is down. When my weight is up I feel heavy like I have weights on me. It's scary. . . . When I don't eat I can't feel my feelings . . . the anguish. . . . It is almost like a buzz . . . just like a high. (Gulley, 1991, p. 112)

My cupboards have never been as full as when I was starving. It's like, see how powerful I am. Look at all this food and I'm not going to eat it. (p. 120)

Winning out over food meant old guilt and inadequacy could be forgotten. They felt high and sought to continue the high by denying rational thoughts:

My rational brain says, the normal body weight for you is this, and you are not fat, but this disease in me says, look here, look there--your thighs just spread out, and your butt, and your stomach. (Gulley, 1991, p. 118)

Double Life

Anorexia and bulimia became private strategies for dealing with all kinds of stress. Isolation and secrecy increased as shame and self-dislike increased. Relationships might be maintained, but true intimacy was avoided, as the real self was unlikeable. For bulimics, a guilt--self-punishment--reward cycle developed, in which tension and distress would build until bingeing brought numbness and purging brought resolution and a return to control. Emotions and interpersonal needs or conflicts could not be expressed to others; they were handled privately as the private rituals of self-care and self-control became increasingly shameful.

What started as friends' admiration for becoming attractively thin turned into concern or rejection as the young women became emaciated. Even when diagnosed with anorexia or bulimia, many women were unable to change, fearing again the powerlessness and self-hate that had been their prior existence. Controlling therapists and rigid behavior modification treatment intensified this resistance in some. What began as the perfect way to be liked and included in life had turned into a lonely battle for control over the hidden needy self.

The Urge to Overeat

Dolhanty (1990) interviewed five young Canadian women struggling with overeating and obsession with food. These women described a split, disengaged sense of self, which they heard as two voices. One was their rational, thinking self, and the other was an irrational, emotive self. The urge to overeat was like an unbearable tension, a growing obsession in which the emotive self took over. Several women likened it to the urge for drugs.

> Like: "I need it." Like: "No, no, don't have it." I'm fighting all the time. It's like two people struggling for control. The way I define it is my rational side versus my emotional side, and the emotional side 99% of the time wins out. (pp. 59-60)

They described being distracted from their school work by preoccupation with their next meal. Efforts at redirecting the urge to eat only postponed the problem. They described feeling that they were going crazy as they fought the urge, and that something terrible would happen if they did to give in to it. From their rational sides, they could cite childhood pain, loneliness, stress, feeling unloved, and low confidence as causes of overeating, yet they rarely could apply this knowledge when under pressure from the emotional self to eat. When they finally ate, they felt that they'd failed, and they might as well go all the way and binge, to get it out of their systems and not do it again. Then the cycle repeated itself.

They ate to help themselves feel better but felt worse when they ate. Eating promised comfort, security, reassurance, and self-nurturing, yet it never succeeded. When recovering from a binge, the pain of self-denial, obsession, and self-hate was enormous, yet the urge to eat overpowered the knowledge that overeating would cause more pain. In a process similar to dissociation, women distanced themselves from that awareness as they gave in to the urge. Sadly, they often could not taste or enjoy the food they ate beyond the first bites. Without the satisfaction of enjoying the food, they never felt they had had enough.

Dolhanty (1990) found that these young women described their whole lives in terms of their weight: when they were thin, when they were heavy, when other pursuits were predominant, and when eating took ascendancy once again. They related the ups and downs of their school work, relationships, and careers to their weight at the time.

But in reality, I don't know who I am, because this is really covering up my real self, the eating is covering up who I am. (p. 91)

Some saw the route to recovery as accepting themselves as fat and letting go of social prescriptions for thinness, and others saw controlling overeating as the goal that would bring stable weight and peace of mind. Yet none had achieved sustained focus on other avenues of life.

Reckoning With Old Pain: Learning to Feel

The eventual goal of recovery from eating disorders is learning to recognize and manage painful feelings without numbing or self-punishment through disordered eating. Persic (1993) interviewed Canadian women with bulimia. They also described a pervasive sense of lack of control in painful, chaotic early lives and buildups of frustration that led to binges and bulimia. One woman described spending $70 for a day's pastries. She kept chewable laxatives in a chewing gum box so they were always accessible (p. 89).

However, several of the older women had begun to find other ways of coping. The voice of the fearful, injured, confused self was coming out despite their best efforts. They found in therapy that when they faced the reality of their pain and accepted that they were not to blame, the bulimia faded a bit. They could begin to seek other ways of coping with their pain, such as looking for information, positive social support, solace in faith and prayer, and professional help. They learned to plan ahead to solve problems to avoid being overwhelmed, and eventually to eat in moderation.

Reconciling With Food: Restructuring Inner Self and Outer Life

Women who overeat without bulimia may also find that they need to examine their beliefs about themselves and change their lifestyles to achieve weight control. Johnson (1990) studied women in a weight-loss program and identified a three-stage process of *restructuring*, in which women first gained a sense of control, then worked on changing their perspectives, and last, integrated a new identity and way of life. As the reader will quickly recognize, these stages resemble other recovery processes as well. In this case, behavior changes occurred before reckoning really began, as a result of the outside influence of the structured weight-loss program.

Gaining a sense of control was begun by reorganizing oneself and the environment. In the early stages, women disciplined themselves with self-imposed distraction or avoidance of food. They made changes in their personal activities and environment to avoid being prompted to eat:

> I'm getting all the things out of the way that I could use for an excuse. I'm not even watching TV very much. . . . TV is loaded with commercials about eating all the wrong things. (Johnson, 1990, p. 1291)

After the program for weight loss was in place, women took initial steps toward coming to terms with self: reflecting on the role of overeating in their lives, realizing that they had alternatives, and committing to action to change their eating.

> I made up my mind . . . I was going to do something for myself. I cut my hair, pierced my ears, and started on a diet. . . . We are responsible for our own attitudes and spirit and can feel in control. (p. 1292)

This internal work increased their self-confidence and trust in themselves, enabling them to rely less on external structures, such as the diet program, and more on their own changing outlook.

The main work of restructuring was changing perspective, reckoning with the roots of unhealthy behavior. The women came to four realizations. The first was that they could meet their own needs, rather than making others' well-being and acceptance a priority. Women began to realize that their hunger was not always a physical need and that they were sometimes looking for other kinds of nurturing and approval when they ate. They made changes in family patterns, friendships, and work situations in which they had been taken advantage of as insecure overweight women. They became more assertive about their own worth.

The second realization was a redefinition of success and failure as they looked at the larger picture of what they were trying to accomplish. They learned over time to view a slip in their diet as a temporary setback rather than failure and to feel more in control and responsible even after episodes of overeating.

> If you are going to go out and . . . eat pizza tonight that does not mean for the next few days you have to eat pizza. (Johnson, 1990, p. 1293).

The third realization was insight into the origins of their eating styles and beliefs about dieting. For many, their childhood family meal experiences had been rushed and competitive. Food was a substitute for communication. The fourth realization was that overeating was a chronic problem and that binge eating might recur; it would always be a possibility.

In the final stage of losing weight, women integrated a new identity and way of life. They tested their limits of flexibility of food intake, finding out how to live with tempting foods rather than avoid them. As women developed a "thin mentality," they had to adjust their beliefs about how being thin would change their lives, as well as come to terms with their new appearances and social acceptability. Successful weight-losers worked to develop ongoing support systems that helped rather than sabotaged their efforts to maintain their weight loss. As the structure of the diet program became less central, women created their own personal routines and built new understandings of others and themselves. The large majority of women attempting weight loss do not succeed. Hamilton (1988) interviewed U. S. women who had lost weight but had varying success in maintaining the loss over time. Women who were successful continually monitored the many factors that influenced eating and weight control. They maintained awareness of how their history, psychological influences, situations, and the presence of food could lead them to overeat. Monitoring also enabled women to confront themselves honestly with the facts about what they were eating and its effects and to support themselves effectively. This internal monitoring had taken the place of the external monitoring previously provided by their weight-loss program. All the women were aware of appropriate options for food and exercise, but women who regained weight were unable or unwilling to monitor themselves and take steps to maintain weight control. They saw themselves as lazy, their old patterns too deep, and healthy food as unenjoyable.

Strategies of successful weight maintainers were geared at planning and organizing resources to promote weight control. They sometimes confronted self and others--assertively refusing pressure to eat and asking for what they needed, and admitting to themselves what they had eaten or wanted to eat. They also supported themselves, planning and rationalizing good choices and meeting their own psychological needs. In contrast, strategies of regainers were aimed at legitimizing their backsliding in eating habits. They were too tired, too busy, one cookie won't hurt, three is not much more than one, and so forth. Legitimizing often included eating as a form of misguided self-care, which (as it did for bulimic women) could lead over time to feelings of despair and hopelessness.

> It tasted good going down. There was an initial rush. I shoved it in and it tasted good. But when it got down into here, I felt terrible. I know it would have been better for me to have one, not have the whole dozen. I felt physically sick to my stomach. (Hamilton, 1988, p. 77)

Learning to eat well could bring feelings of control, as dieting originally did for young girls who became anorexic. With self-knowledge, however, this control could be a positive influence.

> Okay, I ate my celery and my apple, and I had this nice salad and everything. . . . Sure, this cookie might taste good, but on the other end of the spectrum

> I wouldn't feel good about it. I would feel guilty. And over here where I am now, I feel like I am in control of myself and I feel more powerful. (Hamilton, 1988, p. 78)

Women who maintained their weight loss were aware of the psychological influences on their eating and the long-term nature of their overeating problems. The successful maintainers gave up long-held habits of shopping and cooking and began healthier patterns, defended these changes within their families, and found ways to see the good in their new choices. Honesty was a critical component of monitoring and was the opposite of legitimizing. Even for women who monitored themselves less closely, if they could maintain honesty about what they might find when they took a closer look, they were likely to take action to remedy their loosened control.

> I can still fool myself, but I can catch myself sooner. And when I get back on the scale, I know that I was just lying to myself and pretending that all was going well with my weight. (Hamilton, 1988, p. 90)

Regainers were not able or willing to self-correct when they saw the consequences of these choices.

> I lost the weight once, and everybody said I looked so good, and now I am skimming my weight back up to where I was. And I'm asking myself why I am doing it, and I don't know. I haven't looked at it far enough. (p. 91)

Regainers seemed to view the behavior changes during treatment as temporary and seemed not to have internalized or accepted the need to adhere to them for the rest of their lives. They viewed them as externally imposed rules rather than as personal choices. And keeping the excess weight off was less important to them or less clearly linked to positive feelings.

> I became so conscious of food. I made out menus and wrote down everything I ate all day long. All I thought about was food. I didn't enjoy it. I tried for a year or so. And I just had to stop doing it. I decided there were lots of other things I wanted to worry about besides food and eating. (p. 92)

Although successful maintainers did relax their observance at times, they were able to keep the long view, to see the lifelong nature of their tendencies to overeat and to respond to the consequences of their slips. Regainers were unwilling to honestly examine their reasons for overeating and to deal with their negative feelings in other ways.

In sum, reckoning with an eating problem means looking below the food responses to the feelings underneath, often facing sadness and childhood pain, and accepting the reality of self-discipline required to change eating behavior.

Reconciling is the process of finding new ways to nurture oneself and meet needs without resorting to self-destructive behavior. Each of these steps requires intensive work for women severely affected by anorexia or bulimia, and deep-seated childhood experiences often must be uncovered. Then, the problematic family issues must be dealt with in the present as well. At all levels of severity of eating problems, continued honest self-exploration and self-direction is essential to identify and deal with the feelings that lead women to use food or food avoidance to feel better about themselves.

SUBSTANCE ABUSE RECOVERY: SUSTAINING HEALTHY SELF-NURTURING

Rescue or Refuge: Drugs to Shield Vulnerability

Women who develop addictions to alcohol or drugs describe a trajectory somewhat similar to women with eating disorders: a downward slide in which a pattern that at first brings comfort becomes their major preoccupation, a necessity for coping. Indeed, the two problems often occur together, and the core process of recovery involves similar kinds of work.

In this discussion, addiction refers both to alcohol and other legal and illegal substances producing physical or psychological dependency. Yet it must be said that women addicted to alcohol usually are not alienated from mainstream society to the same extent as women primarily addicted to illicit drugs, such as heroin or cocaine. One can drink alcohol quite heavily within many socially accepted contexts, and alcohol is much less expensive than illegal drugs sold in underground economies. Although alcohol certainly destroys health, impairs women's ability to work and relate to others, and can produce job loss and family disintegration, it does not often produce poverty due to the cost of the substance alone, as cocaine can do. And alcohol can be obtained within the legal market; it does not require becoming involved with a network of marginalized, dangerous sellers and users. For these reasons, women addicted to alcohol may be better able than women addicted to illicit drugs to hold together a semblance of normal life.

Illicit drug use can offer mainstream images of success in a marginalized world. Women raised in poverty or in neighborhoods or families already involved in illicit economies gravitate toward the drugs used for recreation in their communities. Furthermore, women who have been victims of racism, crumbling educational systems, and multigenerational economic dependence have little evidence that "straight" life has anything to offer them. They may lack basic skills to build a career and economic security, or harbor resentment of a society that has excluded them. They may have had children as young adolescents and lost hope of "becoming" anything other than a single mother. In such a context, drugs seem a logical alternative, a means of escaping harsh realities, claiming a glittering fast-life identity and doing something nice for oneself (Kearney, Murphy, & Rosenbaum, 1994).

When Woodhouse (1992) studied urban, poor women in a drug treatment center, the women described their lives as chaotic and isolated from sources of stability and routine. As one woman said, "The bizarre is the usual" (p. 270). Early family life had been frightening, painful, and often characterized by substance abuse. Violence and victimization were frequent, and rape was so common as to be considered normal by some women. Male dominance and dependence on men was accepted as necessary and unavoidable. The women had little sense of self-worth outside relationships with men. Isolation from others by violent partners further weakened women's sense of their own value. Many were mothers and had struggled to shield children from the effects of drugs and care for them while trying to pacify and serve the man of the house. They felt unable to see other pathways for themselves and had few skills with which to pursue independence. In their treatment program, stopping drug use was only a small step toward discovering who they could become.

Encountering Drugs

Whether rich or poor, adolescent or middle-aged, women very often become involved in drugs or alcohol abuse in the context of relationships. Early family experiences that are abusive or neglectful, especially when alcohol or drugs are used by parents or role models, can lead young women to rebel or escape in drugs introduced by siblings or peers. A woman often is introduced to drugs by a male partner (Henderson, Boyd, & Mieczkowski, 1994), and her desire to be in the relationship leads to sharing the partner's habit along with other aspects of life. Others seem to overcome early difficulty and are involved in stable lives and successful work when they find that a drug or alcohol fills a space where something is missing. Still others discover the power of drugs when they are prescribed a narcotic to relieve physical pain and find that this relief helps them cope with other stressors as well.

In interviews with ethnically diverse women enrolled in a treatment program for pregnant and parenting women (Kearney, 1996), we found that drugs served originally as rescue or refuge. Many looked back on their entry into drugs as relief from the pain of past or present abuse, and several simply described acute boredom and hopelessness as reasons for the appeal of drugs. This woman started using heroin in high school:

> I was very self-conscious, I was awkward as a child, and drugs made those feelings go away, they made me feel good enough. It solved all my problems, it felt like. (p. 763)

Another woman said, "I just did it mostly to fit in . . . to feel loved by somebody" (p. 764).

Native American women alcohol users (Lowery, 1994) described the trauma they had encountered as children as multigenerational, stemming from the violent disenfranchisement, forced labor, geographic and family dislocation, murder by epidemic, and cultural annihilation of their peoples by white Americans. All had parents who used alcohol, and all had grown up with one or both parents unavailable to them. Many had been victims of violence or abuse, and all the women had abused their own children. The pain their families felt and passed on to them was experienced as both situational and spiritual. Alcoholism was viewed as a loss of spiritual connection and harmony, an alienation from traditional values of gratitude and reciprocity. The women's grandparents had known something of traditional tribal life, but by the time their parents were having children, anomie and violence were the norm. Many felt deep anger at their mothers for not protecting them as children, for not carrying on the responsibility and power accorded to women in their Indian tradition, and for submitting to domination by alcohol, whites, and men. With little economic opportunity and no sense of purpose, the Native American women became heavy drinkers in their teens and continued in drinking, violence, and skirmishes with the law through their childbearing years.

In a study of chemically dependent nurses, Hutchinson (1986) found that the nurses were also suffering from psychic and physical pain: One reported, "I suffer from migraines and chronic backaches that interfere with every aspect of my life." Another stated, "I am totally overworked and have no back-up support. They give me responsibility but no authority. I feel impotent" (p. 198). Some discovered drugs by self-medication or misuse of prescription pain medications; others were initiated into drug use in recreational contexts or with intimate partners. When they connected the drug use with a great deal of relief, they began experimenting with types and amounts of drugs, seeking a way to achieve that relief while maintaining their work and other activities.

When drugs became essential, either due to physical addiction or psychological dependency, nurses conducted a dialog with themselves, justifying the drug use as necessary, bargaining with themselves to set limits on how far they would go to obtain drugs, and denying that their drug use was a serious problem. Like women with eating problems, they began to disengage from aspects of themselves: their consciences, their awareness of what was really going on, and their usual behavior and interactions. This enabled them to enter an outsider role, a deviant lifestyle as a drug user, and escape scrutiny by significant others.

I withdrew more and more from my family and friends. I would not let anyone help me or get to me. In a way I became a totally different person. I was totally into myself. (Hutchinson, 1986, p. 199)

As drinking or drug use became a daily routine and nurses began to deceive themselves about their habit, they also developed strategies to deceive others in order to obtain and use drugs or alcohol without detection. Last, they reached the stage of compulsion, when craving drove their daily life. They lost all support except from accomplices in deception, were in serious trouble at work, and eventually faced criminal prosecution or loss of their nursing licenses, yet these losses were minimized or numbed by self-deception and continued use of drugs.

Hitting Bottom and Surrendering: Reckoning With Addiction

Many recovery stories involve "hitting bottom," suddenly reaching a point where the only way to survive was to give up alcohol or drugs, but women also describe gradual awakenings to their problems with addiction. Hall (1994) studied ethnically diverse lesbian women with alcohol problems. They reported that awareness of their addiction problem could be sudden, such as being arrested, or more long term, such as growing awareness that one was drinking heavily as a response to discrimination. Some found indicators within themselves. "Inside I couldn't stand what I had become, even though no one was criticizing any of these things about me" (p. 52).

Hutchinson (1987) also found that a critical juncture led nurses into recovery and could be triggered by either external or internal pressure. One nurse described an internal realization that she was "hitting the bottom of the barrel":

> My daughter was about to be taken from me by the child protection team. My alimony was over. I had been stolen from, abused, and in fights. I couldn't remember what I did from day to day. I had been hospitalized from numerous car accidents and had lost my license. I knew I would die if I didn't stop drinking and drugging. (p. 340)

Native American women also reached a point of intolerable incongruence between their views of themselves and their traditional beliefs, although those beliefs were sometimes deeply submerged and not brought back to awareness until a crisis occurred. This woman found herself being promiscuous:

> I had to look at myself and say, "this is going too far." . . . I felt like I dishonored myself . . . that's not what I am. And I would always feel really . . . disgusted with myself. Like I'd really . . . done something wrong, or done something bad for myself, for my spirit. (Lowery, 1994, p. 62)

For addicted women in a variety of social contexts, threats to their loved ones prompted new awareness of their problem. Some who had given up on themselves as worth saving found they could not fail their children.

Obstacles to Seeking Help

Despite serious consequences, many women continue drug or alcohol use long after they realize something is wrong or others have recognized their problems and urged them to seek help. Beyond "denial," many powerful forces prevent women from taking steps to confront the problem even after they have recognized its seriousness. Life in a multigenerational drinking culture prevented Native American women from readily identifying other ways of life as accessible or normal (Lowery, 1994). Many nurses were able to continue working and functioning while using drugs by using their professional knowledge and status to obtain drugs, convincing themselves that they were taking reasonable actions (Hutchinson, 1986).

Hall (1994) identified perceptual constraints, including women's beliefs that they were different from real alcoholics or addicts, reluctance to face the deep emotional roots of their drinking, and dissociation as a result of childhood and adult trauma.

I didn't want to think of myself as needing help. . . . I had never had a DWI [driving while intoxicated]. Never been to jail. I mean I had heard all these stories. And they all got filtered through this image of myself as the responsible citizen. A lesbian businesswoman. (p. 53-54)

Environmental constraints that prevented lesbians from dealing with their alcohol problems included the prevalence of alcohol at lesbian social functions and gathering places, racism and homophobia in helping professionals, lack of insurance or available addiction treatment, barriers to women and homosexuals in treatment settings, the utility of substance abuse to cope with demeaning work and social situations, and opposition of significant others to their seeking help. Like Native American women, this lesbian woman felt unable to disentangle the problems rooted in alcohol from the many other stressors and hurts she was coping with over time:

I didn't know what my options were, financially. I couldn't see that there was anything out there to fix whatever I had. I thought "This isn't a problem, it's just my life." (Hall, 1994, p. 54)

To take action, women had to reach a point where these constraints were overcome by the overwhelming necessity to stop drinking and using drugs. For some, this necessity became apparent suddenly, and others gradually reached a breaking point. Either form of critical juncture could lead a woman to take the frightening first steps toward a new life.

Encountering Honesty

Naming the Problem

Being able to call oneself an alcoholic or an addict is widely seen as the first step toward recovery. For some women, realizing that their overwhelming problems can be attributed to an involuntary "disease" of addiction is a huge relief. Yet, "surrendering" to an identity as an alcoholic requires overcoming a great deal of resistance (Maroni, 1986). It then can be followed by grief, if what had been considered a small temporary problem now has to be redefined as a lifelong burden. This is a moment of honest self-appraisal, and it sets the tone for continued work on truthful self-nurturing.

At first, it can be all a woman can do to simply stay abstinent. Hulbert (1985) studied Canadian women who had been in recovery from 1 to over 6 years. They described how early recovery was characterized by self-protection through withdrawal. Women focused on getting through their days without drinking, and they had no energy left over to risk encountering other people. Many were fearful of others' anger or rejection or were accustomed to isolating themselves to avoid contact with their real selves.

> I was leading two lives because I carried on my job and everything else and you know, here's one image and then there was this other bit of humanity in absolute pain, and I couldn't show that publicly. . . . [The group leaders] accepted me as a friend, even though, at the time, I was incapable of handling it . . . I wasn't able even to feel it or let it touch me. (p. 120-121)

Counselors are familiar with the phenomenon in which women who become clean and sober begin to experience as if for the first time the emotional distress that may have triggered their addiction. This can take the form of depression, grief, anxiety, post-traumatic symptoms, or anger.

> I was terrified, terrified of anger! Even if there was a fracas on the subway, halfway down the car, I would be frightened, as if, somehow, I was responsible. . . . Very distressing to be around any of it, and my own was unthinkable! I didn't feel it for years, and years, and years, and years. (Hulbert, 1985, p. 122).

Hulbert (1985) found that women at this early stage had little sense of their own identity and felt ruled by external events and their emotional reactions to them. Interactions with others often brought distress and temptation to relapse, but being in relationships seemed central to being oneself. Women were reluctant to pull away from long-standing ties, even when those ties were abusive. Women often distracted themselves from their own pain and bolstered shaky self-worth by focusing on giving to others and self-sacrifice (p. 146). Chemically dependent nurses described surrendering to the reality of their addiction: acknowledging to themselves and others that they were addicted, confessing to the harms they had caused in pursuit of chemicals, and simply praying for continued sobriety, tactics learned in Alcoholics Anonymous (AA) and personalized by the women over time (Hutchinson, 1987). They worked to accept addiction as a part of themselves, with the faults and failings that being an addict implied. The disease model of addiction was readily accepted by nurses, who could accept an identity as someone with an illness more easily than as someone with a behavioral problem.

Abstinence as an Inadequate Solution

As women strengthened their skills of avoiding substance abuse, they began to learn about themselves in new ways and to see other areas of needed change. Until they embarked on personal growth, they were often stuck, "leaving drugs but not the drug life" (Kearney, 1996), continuing old self-defeating patterns. Their problems and often the solutions were seen as outside themselves. A substance abuse counselor reported that women who had been unable to move forward despite achieving abstinence would tell her they were bored, didn't trust anybody, weren't doing anything or making any changes, yet wondered why their lives weren't getting any better. Relapses were common. Only women who were convinced that abstinence was essential for their futures reached the difficult conclusion that something even larger was at stake and their present strategies weren't working. Then, they began to participate more fully in their treatment.

Vourakis (1989) also found that as women worked to maintain sobriety over time, they increasingly saw the need for personal growth work in addition to abstinence work, and they became more discriminating about the AA meetings they attended. They began to build important relationships with people in these meetings and attended fewer groups, choosing those in which they felt safe and supported as their participation increased.

Reconciling: Toward Self-Integration

Hutchinson (1987) described self-integration in nurses' recovery as reclaiming wholeness and self-worth. This internal reweaving of physical, psychological, social, philosophical, and spiritual integrity required a commitment to a new life. Nurses began to think in new ways about themselves and try on new actions as they returned to their lives. At first, they simply went through the motions of abstinence without faith in their effectiveness.

Eventually, they began to live more honestly with themselves and others and find new ways of nurturing themselves.

Pregnant and parenting drug users had an even longer road to climb to rebuild normal life, as many had never experienced stability and self-sufficiency (Kearney, 1996). Accustomed to protecting themselves from a harsh world, women shielded their self-concepts from suggestions for change. Yet some eventually experienced a distinct transition that their counselors labeled "clearing up," in which these women came to realize that recovery involved restructuring in many areas. This realization brought a major change in their outlook and enjoyment of life. Simple tasks became important steps toward reclaiming normal life.

> It feels so good normal. Getting up in the morning and having a list of things that I want to do, things that I didn't want to do before, clean the bathroom, do laundry. . . . It's neat, 'cause there's a lot of pleasure in doing that stuff that you bitched about before. (p. 765)

Once this realization had occurred, women could reject their abusive boyfriends, disengage from old social groups, work hard in therapy, and refocus their energy beyond avoiding drugs to what they wanted out of life. An initial exhilaration was often followed by depression and struggle, but women had a clearer view of what work lay ahead and what they could hope to achieve by persisting. Many of these urban poor women had to start from scratch to finish their educations, learn employable skills, find new ways of relating to their children and significant others, and cope with setbacks and frustrations. Treatment professionals became crucially important as guides to healthy but unfamiliar relationships and behaviors.

A similar transition was described by Hulbert (1985) as alcoholic women moved from other-centered existence as a way of defining themselves to finding connectedness in equality with others. Women came to see that giving was most rewarding when it arose from equality without sacrifice of self. They realized that conflict was sometimes necessary to preserve selfhood and meet their own needs. They became more comfortable with getting help and more able to relax and be playful. They began to see inequality in wider society and to challenge social expectations for women's dependency and submission.

Maroni (1986) described later alcoholism recovery as strengthening of self, internalizing life changes, and ultimately transcending immediate experience to a broad understanding of meaning and purpose in life.

> Now, I have some understanding of who I am and what I am and where I need to make some changes in me. That's where I am today--and that's growth, and maybe that's dealing with my alcoholism. I really believe that if I don't change those old thinking patterns, I'll get drunk again. (p. 90)

These women became active participants in recovery, taking initiative to monitor themselves and analyze problems, at the same time recognizing that they still needed outside help to remain sober. They became increasingly aware of situations that could trigger vulnerability, including joyous times as well as difficult ones:

> I was out there on the porch with my family having a wonderful time. All of a sudden the lake looked beautiful and this amazing thought came in with the wind saying, "Boy, wouldn't it be nice to have a drink?" . . . I then realized the happy times could be more difficult than the sad times. I feel far more vulnerable at times like this. (p. 95)

Women became able to integrate their emotions and their thoughts, were more skillful at perceiving their vulnerability, and took responsibility for working toward their goals.

> I feel better when I'm moving in the direction of better health and better attitudes. It's a matter of choice. It comes down to taking responsibility. (Maroni, 1986, p. 99)

They developed a "common sense framework " (p. 103) to manage challenges of daily living, and tapped into their own capacities for love and generosity from a newfound position of strength.

> Going through the pain created a lot of depth in me--a lot of compassion and love. To me there is no limit to what can happen. (p. 102)

Native American women (Lowery, 1994) experienced healing from addiction as strengthening the spirit. They began hearing messages pushing them toward sobriety, retraced their path into addiction with new awareness, and committed to self-worth and personal goals. In their families and communities, women focused on "expanding the circle," reawakening their spirit through interpersonal connections. They also found themselves "reclaiming the mother," acknowledging the reality of their past hurts but also empathizing with their past caretakers as caught in dismal life situations. Women sought a sense of justice and balance in these reflections and worked to understand their own roles as mothers and caretakers in relation to previous generations.

They grieved for lost opportunities to connect with spiritual traditions in the anger and chaos of their childhoods and began to see that their own mothers had lost this as well. Through peacemaking with family and community, they were freed to nurture themselves. They recognized how their lives fit into history and the future of the community and tribe. They sought to right the imbalance of three generations, finding ways to contribute their rediscovered strength to local tribal groups and family roles. A Yakima woman summed up her reclaiming of her rightful role, albeit late in life:

> I am coming from puberty to womanhood to know who I am inside finally... As an Indian woman at 52, I'm an elder and I need to look at who I am. Because people come to me to be taught. . . . The page has now been turned; the autumn has started to come to spring, even though the twilight years are here. My autumns, I can see them now, and I can feel and I can see my color now. This is me . . . . Other native people will understand what I am talking about. And a lot of times [they're] the only ones that count for me. . . . [I] can be there as a teacher and a leader in terms of just being who I am. (Lowery, 1994, p. 152)

SUPPORTING RECOVERY FROM PROBLEM BEHAVIORS

Women with eating disorders and women with addictions share the experiences of being denied early evidence of self-worth and of having developed logical but harmful ways of avoiding painful truths and soothing frightening emotions. Those who recover, who are moving past these disorders, achieve truthful self-nurturing--the ability to see their life situations, pasts, and feelings more clearly, and take responsibility for relating to others equitably and honestly in order to meet their own needs. These appear to be the tasks of therapy.

The first hard truth women face in reckoning with addiction or an eating disorder is that they have such a problem. Building trust and consistency are essential for counselors as women dance in and out of help-seeking, aware that something is wrong but fearful they don't have the strength or resources for the work required to change. Counselors are called on to be supportive yet truthful, to set limits on their own time but not on their belief in each woman's potential for change. Many months or years may pass before a troubled woman comes to accept her need for help and the depth of her issues, but her presence in treatment, whether continuous or intermittent, indicates awareness of pain and desire for change.

Women's stories reveal that concrete behavioral techniques and cognitive-behavioral relapse prevention are useful in early recovery, when women have little awareness of what leads them to relapse or little confidence in their ability to stay "clean" and out of trouble on their own. Group work on recognizing stressors and triggers for slipping into old patterns, and distraction or avoidance strategies to prevent relapse, can build confidence in early months. Simply filling hours of the day with work, meetings, and activities is important in early weeks. Contingency and reward systems and structured levels of privileges also have been somewhat effective.

Firm guidance by peers in self-help groups and sponsorship by experienced members is especially useful early on. Yet just as for abused women, controlling or paternalistic tactics in therapy may replicate past abuse and push addicted women away from help. Clients must frequently revisit their commitments to change if they are to participate in a fully voluntary manner. Counselors must have clear consent and support of clients in imposing structures. An obvious complication is legally mandated treatment. For some women, 6 months of mandated treatment can lead to a lasting commitment to change, but unfortunately, for many, it is only a taste of success that at best may bring them back voluntarily sometime in the future.

Many women in addiction treatment move from cognitive-behavioral techniques toward more insight-oriented therapy. However, some women may start in psychotherapy for their emotional distress and then gain strength to examine their addiction. Both addicted women and those who are in the process of losing excess weight start by building minimal levels of confidence that they can survive for a period of time away from their problematic behavior. Eventually, continued unhappiness, anxiety, or frustration will lead women committed to treatment to take risks and examine deeper issues. There will likely be periods of relapse as they struggle to accept the need for this difficult work.

In addition to reckoning with the reality of a behavioral problem, women must reckon with the experiences underneath these propensities, whether family trauma, cultural or social oppression, or other sources of pain. Women also need to learn honest self-awareness in the present. Over time, women can learn to link current feelings and actions to long-standing issues. Life history reviews, either written or in therapeutic dialog; journals; workbooks; prayer and meditation; group work; and self-help groups can be useful. The goal of insight is honest self-appraisal, yet 12-step programs in which one conducts personal inventories may work best later in treatment rather than in early weeks when women have little confidence in their own insight.

To reconcile with the work of continuing recovery from behavioral problems, women must learn to respond to their stressors, thoughts, and emotions in self-nurturing ways. In early weeks of therapy, counselors can provide role-modeling as they demonstrate healthy life patterns and provide appropriate nurturing to clients. Women can be included in tasks, group projects, and recreation that bring satisfaction and boost self-worth. Counselors can work with women to examine how they take care of themselves physically and psychologically. They can work on recognizing and maintaining interpersonal boundaries, managing criticism, coping with frustration and loss, dealing with vulnerability and love relationships, and fostering emotional self-sufficiency.

Counselors can encourage women to explore their personal spiritual leadings. Religious settings may provide a supportive place where acceptance of one's failings and asking for ongoing strength are part of a worship ritual. Pastoral counseling or religious retreats may allow for self-examination and self-nurturing. When it appears that a woman is rushing into a rigid religious tradition with restrictive social mores, counselors may be tempted to discredit this as revictimization or misplaced "surrender." Yet religion may be a socially sanctioned source of external structure that serves as a bridge to deeper self-understanding and eventual self-control.

Counselors can work with women to discern whether practices developed as a means of rebuilding a life without substances increase self-awareness and healthy self-nurturing or deny the primacy of women's selfhood. This is a long-term process, as women are often starting over as they attempt to structure the relationships and self-appraisals of normal living. In the course of therapy, women can be helped to judge emerging life commitments in light of their growing understandings of who they are and the goals they have set.

Normalizing life in the aftermath of an eating or substance abuse disorder means (as in chronic illness) giving up the notion that life ever will be truly spontaneous and carefree. The constant monitoring described by successful weight losers will be needed by recovering addicts as well. The potential reward is a sense of harmony and empowerment, as women begin to internalize the ability to feel, advocate for, and meet their own needs.

8

Supporting Women Toward Health

Future Directions

BUILDING ON THEORIES OF WOMEN AND HEALTH

Ideas about healing are worthy products in themselves, when they sensitize helpers to the issues facing women who embark on a substantial recovery process. But it remains to be determined how best to apply the tools of the counseling profession to aid women who become stuck at points along the way. A great deal more research is needed to demonstrate how these steps can best be facilitated.

We still need to hear the stories of women in the shadows, those not tapped for the research described in this book. Other illness conditions should be looked at and reference materials developed that bring together biomedical and social facts about diseases with women's experiences of their effects. Much more "hard science" medical research is needed to determine women's responses to the many therapies that have been tested only on men but are then applied to women in treatment settings. Counseling protocols must be tested to determine the best combinations of therapeutic techniques for women in various illness situations. This work has begun for conditions such as anorexia and post-traumatic stress but now must branch out to help women with biophysical diseases. For example, the simple finding in one study that support groups are not as effective as cognitive skills training in relieving depression for women with cancer (Telch & Telch, 1986) is the kind of information that should be validated and expanded to women in other health crises.

MISSING PIECES FOR FUTURE RESEARCH

Many questions can be raised about the best formats for treatment. Perhaps, support groups need to be tailored to stages of adjustment to illness, as has been suggested by Herman (1992) for stages of recovery from trauma and is common in addiction recovery programs. It may well be that newly diagnosed women can benefit from a different kind of group than veterans with chronic disease. Or perhaps peer support of "newcomers" through phone calls would fit better than scheduled groups into their still-active lifestyles. Perhaps counseling contact could be built into the health care process at key transition points of illness, such as during diagnosis, at the end of treatment when remission is evaluated, or when cancer recurs, diabetes begins to affect eyesight, or MS flares up.

In another example, given that women with chronic pain repeatedly and unsuccessfully seek medication or solutions from health care providers until they have reckoned with their ongoing burden, counselors with expertise in this area could develop and test "chronic pain support guidelines" for physicians. Such a protocol might identify some of the key issues in working with these women, suggest when and how to refer to counseling, and outline the alternative treatment approaches that have been found effective (including but not limited to mind-body approaches and other modalities offered in chronic pain specialty clinics). Physicians are not trained to foster empowerment. Until such guidelines are commonly available, health care providers are less likely to move beyond the paradigm of using drugs to fix symptoms toward professional support for women's self-management, and women will continue to be medicated with sedating and addictive narcotics and be made to feel that they are mentally unstable, shamefully needy, or hopeless.

More focused study is needed on those women who even after prolonged counseling work are unable to reckon with or become reconciled to their illness conditions. When the kinds of life situations and personal backgrounds that create such difficulties are identified, special effort can be made to identify these women early and offer more intensive support. This will be a cost-saving project in the long run. For example, women with diabetes incur great health care costs due to complications of the illness, such as heart disease, kidney failure, and blindness. To the degree that preventive self-care can reduce the incidence of these complications, early identification and counseling support of women who are stuck in what Armstrong (1990) termed a frustration-cheat-repent cycle may save them great suffering and early loss of life and reduce the huge health care expenditures on diabetes complications.

Another need for study lies in the area of substance abuse recovery. Studies reviewed in this book support the importance of moving beyond abstinence to more pervasive life change if women are to successfully recover from addiction, yet abstinence remains the criterion for recovery in many structured programs. Some women with long-term resistance to standard treatments may need to approach substance abuse recovery from alternate directions: focusing on self-awareness work and relationship changes before they can seriously look at abstinence. Substance abuse counseling services must develop and test ways of assessing women's readiness for these different areas of focus in order to tailor recovery programs to individual needs. The same goes for overeating: Some women achieve weight control only after recognizing and changing deep-seated patterns of self-regard and relating to others, whereas others can find the strength to examine these issues only after the success of losing weight. More work is needed to develop ways of identifying and reaching women with different priorities for change and nurturing them on their own pathways of reckoning and reconciling.

In heart disease, the biggest killer of postmenopausal women, much work still is needed. Clearly, health professionals are not yet successfully conveying the message to women that heart disease is their greatest risk and that it is a chronic and progressive condition more life-threatening than cancer. For women to reckon with the real threats of heart disease early in its course, counseling input is needed very early in the treatment and rehabilitation process, before many women drop out or begin to lose interest in the behavior focused messages of many rehabilitation programs. Women must reckon with the life-threatening and chronic nature of their conditions before they can become reconciled to the need for lifelong health monitoring and behavioral change. As long as health care providers convey the message that this is a man's disease and that it is curable by medical intervention, women will continue to die after heart attacks at a greater rate than men.

HELPING WOMEN TALK THROUGH ILLNESS

In the meantime, while research continues into better ways of identifying women at risk and supporting women through serious illness and trauma, counselors can use the experiences of women described and quoted in this book as fuel for sensitive and individualized work with clients. Counselors must respect the importance to women of being heard as they tell their stories: of presenting the start, middle, and end of an illness experience as a way of conveying meaning (DeVault, 1990). Modification of the routine counseling intake may be important so as to hear women's critical issues as they face illness in their lives, as often these issues can only be conveyed through narrative and exemplar (Munhall & Boyd, 1993).

This is not to say that long-standing skills and techniques should be abandoned in favor of having women run their own counseling sessions; rather, it is simply a reminder that as expert clinicians, we often anticipate the ends of sentences and the conclusions of stories we have heard many times in different forms. Women isolated by pain and suffering are eager for their own realities to be heard and appreciated yet, understandably, doubt that such sharing is possible. The first counseling encounter is often the point at which they decide whether they will be able to bring their illness burdens out into the open and receive help from a respectful and supportive professional.

Counseling help is rarely the first stop in the search for support by a woman facing illness. Her first recourse is usually the health care professionals who provide treatment for the disease condition and her family and intimate friends. When she finally arrives at the counselor's door, it may be at a point of doubt, desperation, or defeat. She may doubt the value of counseling when, in her view, what she faces is a physical problem. She may be desperate for physical relief from symptoms that the medical professionals have been unable to relieve. She may have given up hope that there is any way to survive and grow in the face of a chronic debilitating condition. She may indeed think that she has been labeled as mentally ill due to her unwillingness to live cheerfully with her diminished state.

Counselors thus have the task of conveying to distressed, ill women the tools they have to offer. They must demonstrate their expertise at working not only on day-to-day coping but on larger areas, such as identity shifts and social adjustment. They can share resources such as connections with sources of alternative therapy, peer support groups, useful literature, and sometimes, more compatible medical care providers. And most important, they must communicate respect for women's hard-earned sense of self and recognition of the great pain brought on by relinquishing parts of that self to illness and change. A therapeutic partnership in which women are supported as they set their own goals for life with illness and trauma includes grounding in the process of reckoning and reconciling, with its various pitfalls and variations, and faith in human resilience and self-determination.

DIRECTIONS FOR HEALTH CARE AND PUBLIC POLICY

As Thorne (1993), Strauss and Corbin (1988), and others have eloquently demonstrated, the U. S. health care system is clearly designed for acute, self-limiting disease care and not for chronic conditions or ongoing mental illness. Although acknowledging the complex and multilayered nature of cultural, social, and economic systems, Thorne (1993, p. 207) noted that patients are not well served by bureaucratic rules and structures that reduce their self-determination within the system. Individualization of care is essential to effective treatment, as one young patient remarked:

> Well, if they just used their heads sometimes . . . rather than just going straight by the book, kind of thing. Just a little common sense would go a long way--like listening to the patient. And you know, the doctor isn't always right. Every time he says something, it doesn't mean it's gospel. (p. 209)

Strauss and Corbin (1988) suggested that care of chronic illness should be centered in the home rather than the hospital or clinic because this is the arena where ongoing management of the illness takes place. Hospitalization for less than acute exacerbations disrupts effective patterns of care. They advocate for chronic illness care that is a tightly linked partnership between health care professionals and the patient and family, in which the patient is viewed as the expert in her own unique illness situation and the goal is not only treating the disease but optimizing the individual's personally defined quality of life.

Thorne (1993) also noted the importance of coordinating multiple services and systems within the wider system, as women suffering from chronic illnesses often must consult a variety of specialists, who may in turn provide conflicting advice or even potentially dangerous combinations of medications. Involvement of the patient in a team approach with free flow of communication among professionals is important, although such communication must respect patient confidentiality. Another obstacle to effective care is the reimbursement system. Insurer control over what services are offered to patients has increased to the point that legislation has been the only way to ensure minimal standards of service. Counselors can join with other health professionals in calling for individualized needs assessment and humane levels of financial support for care.

Thorne (1993) found that many patients wished for some professional individual who could act as a go-between or advocate to help them navigate the health care system. After years of living with chronic illness, the patients' goal was to be more in charge of their own care. There may be settings in which counselors can function in this advocate role or create such a role. To this end, helpers can increase their knowledge of how the system works and the resources within it by linking with other professionals across the system, learning the particulars of health care payment schemes outside the realm of mental health, and listening to women about who has helped them and what obstacles they have encountered in their search for care.

As Thorne (1993), Kleinman (1988), and others have noted, until very recently medical care systems have been reluctant to respect or take seriously the nonmedical aspects of illness, that is, the psychological, emotional, and social impacts of disease. Counseling, home nursing care, respite care to relieve family caregivers, and other forms of help beyond medical treatment have been poorly funded and difficult to access. Although many counselors are adept at justifying and obtaining payment for their services through creative means, to more fully support women trying to juggle lives around illness, counselors must advocate for access to these other forms of support as well.

Furthermore, medical care systems have been poorly informed about and even more poorly connected with sources of alternative treatment, including traditional Native American healing, Chinese medicine, meditation, spiritual approaches, and even behavioral approaches within mainstream health care. It is often only at the request of a well-informed patient that a referral is made or an alternative approach condoned. When patients seek multiple sources of care simultaneously, they risk dangerous interactions of medications or treatments unless they feel comfortable discussing these combinations with medical professionals.

Counselors may be in the middle of such conflicts, hearing from women about the needs that doctors cannot meet for which they are seeking help from nontraditional sources. Helpers must become knowledgeable not only about the types of therapies available but the principles behind them and the local options for obtaining them safely and appropriately. Much of this knowledge is typically gained from patients themselves, women who have discovered such treatments through trial and error. Much new literature on alternative therapies has emerged for the public and health care providers, and this information can be used by counselors as well.

Marginalization of women on the basis of sex, race, ethnicity, economic status, and sexual orientation remains perhaps the most important obstacle to effective multidisciplinary health care. Although they consume more health care than men, because women still lack power and credibility in many arenas of resource distribution they are only beginning to have control over how that care is administered. Racial and ethnic discrimination has at least in part contributed to the dramatically poorer health status of women and children of color in the United States (Bayne-Smith, 1996). Furthermore, comparatively few health professionals or researchers are of nonwhite race or non-European ethnicity, contributing to the dearth of scientific research on issues important to marginalized groups. Explanations such as blaming the victims of poor health for their unhealthy behaviors deny the real impact of poverty on women's abilities to live healthy lives. The pain of stigmatization for their lack of education, language barriers, or sexual orientation and others' lack of understanding or respect for different cultural beliefs about illness and treatment keeps many needy women away from sources of help, which in turn perpetuates professionals' lack of knowledge of how to help effectively.

One sixth of women in the United States are estimated to have physical and perceptual disabilities, and they represent one of the most invisible minority groups. Disabled women face the same sexism as their able-bodied sisters but are denied the "pedestal" or gender-related rewards granted women who meet accepted standards of beauty (Asch & Fine, 1988). Women with permanent physical challenges often are seen as childlike, asexual, diminished in their capacities, and mentally deficient. The diversity of disabled women's cultures, talents and abilities is easily overshadowed by reactions to the disability itself. At times, feminist activists have left disabled women behind in order to present an image of strength and competence (Asch & Fine, 1988). The progress of rights to access, housing, work, and legal equity for the disabled has been achieved almost exclusively through their own grass-roots efforts. Counselors play a key role in supporting and advocating for disabled women through not only their physical and emotional challenges but the much larger social and legal obstacles they face.

The women's health movement has provided a critically important platform for progress in many arenas of policy change. The vast social impact of the Boston Women's Health Book Collective and their landmark book, *Our Bodies, Ourselves* (e.g., 1985), cannot be underestimated, and concurrent efforts by women in many segments of society have brought women's sensibilities and needs in health care into even the most resistant arenas of health care delivery. The concept of self-help and advocacy for self in health care has crossed gender lines to make patients' rights an expectation in all health care settings.

The consciousness-raising and gains achieved by well-educated white middle-class women still have not trickled down on a personal level to many less advantaged women. Only through empowered women's constant attention to the impact of health policy on women's well-being will the needs of the least visible and vocal women be met. Counselors can provide bridges to empowerment for clients as individuals and underserved women as a group through persistent work toward small-scale changes at personal and local levels, and by advocacy in larger arenas through professional and political action.

Counselors have the skills to hear the voices and needs of women from all backgrounds, and they have the professional status to speak in favor of equity in health care resources. The United States has been called on by Bayne-Smith (1996) and others to make a real investment in women, particularly poor women, in the form not only of financial support for education, job training and restructuring, child care, safety, and health care, but also in legislative priority setting that favors the well-being of women and children as essential to a stable and productive society.

Effort is needed on many fronts to bring this goal into being, but we learn from women's experiences of reckoning and reconciling with illness that one must see and come to terms with unpleasant realities and inequities to move forward toward a better life. When helping professionals internalize the facts of racial, social, and financial inequity and become involved in supporting women who have been harmed by that reality, the voices of women will become louder through their helpers' advocacy, and professionals themselves will be enriched.

References

Allen, J., & Blumenthal, R. (1998). Risk factors in the offspring of women with premature coronary heart disease. *American Heart Journal, 135,* 428-434.

Anderson, C. (1993). *Women's stories on growing up with a father who abused alcohol: Adding new distinctions.* Unpublished masters thesis, University of Guelph, Guelph, Ontario, Canada.

Anderson, D., Ellenberg, G., Leventhal, C., Reingold, S., Rodriguez, M., & Silverberg, H. (1992). Revised estimate of the prevalence of multiple sclerosis in the United States. *Annals of Neurology, 31,* 333-336.

Angell, M. (1993). Caring for women's health: What is the problem? (Editorial). *The New England Journal of Medicine, 329,* 271-272.

Annas, G. (1994). Women, health care, and the law: Birth, death, and in between. In E. Friedman (Ed.), *An unfinished revolution: Women and health care in America,* pp. 29-45. New York: United Hospital Fund of New York.

Armstrong, N. (1987). Coping with diabetes mellitus: A full-time job. *Nursing Clinics of North America, 22,* 559-568.

Armstrong, N. (1990). *Perceptions of adults with insulin-requiring diabetes of factors influencing their self-management.* Unpublished dissertation, University of Georgia, Athens, Georgia.

Asch, A., & Fine, M. (1988). Introduction: Beyond pedestals. In M. Fine and A. Asch (Eds.), *Women with disabilities: Essays in psychology, culture, and politics,* pp. 1-37. Philadelphia: Temple University.

Barrett-Connor, E., & Wingard, D. (1984). Sex differences in diabetes mellitus. In E. Gold (Ed.), *The changing risk of disease in women,* pp. 257-286. Lexington, MA: Heath.

Bayne-Smith, M. (Ed.). (1996). *Race, gender, and health.* Thousand Oaks, CA: Sage.

Belenky, M. (1997). *Women's ways of knowing: The development of self, voice, and mind.* New York: BasicBooks.

Berman, A. (1993). *Sailing a course through chemotherapy: The experience of women with breast cancer.* Unpublished dissertation, University of California at San Francisco.

Boston Women's Health Book Collective. (1985). *The new our bodies, ourselves* (2nd ed., rev.). New York: Simon & Schuster.

Callaghan, D., & Williams, A. (1994). Living with diabetes: Issues for nursing practice. *Journal of Advanced Nursing, 20,* 132-139.

Carlton, S. (1992). *Women's experience of childhood sexual abuse and subsequent development of bulimia nervosa: A grounded theory exploration.* Unpublished dissertation, University of Calgary, Alberta, Canada.

Centers for Disease Control and Prevention. (1994). *Recent trends in reported US AIDS cases.* Atlanta, GA: Author.
Centers for Disease Control and Prevention. (1995). *Facts about women and HIV/AIDS.* Atlanta, GA: Author.
Charmaz, K. (1980). The social construction of self-pity in the chronically ill. *Studies in Symbolic Interaction, 3,* 123-145.
Charmaz, K. (1983). Loss of self: A fundamental form of suffering in the chronically ill. *Sociology of Health and Illness, 5,* 168-195.
Charmaz, K. (1991). *Good days, bad days: The self in chronic illness and time.* New Brunswick, NJ: Rutgers University Press.
Charmaz, K. (1995). The body, identity, and self: Adapting to impairment. *Sociological Quarterly, 36,* 657-680.
Cochrane, B. (1992). *Women's integration of the myocardial infarction experience: Reclaiming independence after a heart attack.* Unpublished dissertation, University of Washington, Seattle.
Constable, D. (1994). *The process of recovery for adult survivors of childhood sexual abuse: A grounded theory study.* Unpublished dissertation, University of Alberta, Edmonton, Alberta, Canada.
Corbin, J., & Strauss, A. (1988). *Unending work and care: Managing chronic illness at home.* San Francisco: Jossey-Bass.
Davis, T., & Jensen, L. (1988). Identifying depression in medical patients. *Image: Journal of Nursing Scholarship, 20,* 191-195.
Dempsey, S., Dracup, K., & Moser, D. (1995). Women's decision to seek care for the symptoms of acute myocardial infarction. *Heart & Lung, 24,* 444-456.
DeVault, M. (1990). Talking and listening from women's standpoint: Feminist strategies for interviewing and analysis. *Social Problems, 37,* 96-116.
Dildy, S. (1992). *A naturalistic study of the nature, meaning and impact of suffering in people with rheumatoid arthritis.* Unpublished dissertation, University of Texas at Austin.
Dildy, S. (1996). Suffering in people with rheumatoid arthritis. *Applied Nursing Research, 9,* 177-183.
Dolhanty, J. (1990). *The urge to overeat: A qualitative analysis of personal accounts.* Unpublished masters thesis, York University Graduate Programme in Psychology, North York, Ontario, Canada.
Dow, K. H. (1994). Having children after breast cancer. *Cancer Practice, 2,* 407-413.
Draucker, C. (1991). The healing process of female adult incest survivors: Constructing a personal residence. *Image: Journal of Nursing Scholarship, 24,* 4-8.
Draucker, C. (1997). Early family life and victimization in the lives of women. *Research in Nursing & Health, 20,* 399-412.
Eagan, A. (1994). The women's health movement and its lasting impact. In E. Friedman (Ed.), *An unfinished revolution: Women and health care in America,* pp. 15-27. New York: United Hospital Fund of New York.
Edelstein, L. (1994). *Maternal bereavement: Coping with the unexpected death of a child.* New York: Praeger.
Ehrenreich, B., & English, D. (1977). Complaints and disorders: The sexual politics of sickness. In C. Dreifus (Ed.), *Seizing our bodies: The politics of women's health,* pp. 43-56. New York: Vintage Books.
Fitzgerald, M., & Paterson, K. (1995). The hidden disability dilemma for the preservation of self. *Journal of Occupational Science, Australia, 2,* 13-21.
Fleury, J., Kimbrell, C., & Kruszewski, M. (1995). Life after a cardiac event:

Women's experience in healing. *Heart & Lung, 24,* 474-482.

Folden, S. (1994). Managing the effects of a stroke: The first months. *Rehabilitation Nursing Research, 3,* 79-85.

Friedman, E. (1994). Women and health care: The bramble and the rose. In E. Friedman (Ed.), *An unfinished revolution: Women and health care in America,* pp. 1-12. New York: United Hospital Fund of New York.

Fuchs, C. (1999). Dietary fiber and the risk of colorectal cancer and adenoma in women.*The New England Journal of Medicine, 340,* 169-176.

Gamble, V., & Blustein, B. (1994). Racial differentials in medical care: Implications for research on women. In A. Mastroianni, R. Faden, & D. Federman (Eds.), *Women and health research: Vol. 2. Workshop and commissioned papers.* Washington, DC: National Academy Press, Institute of Medicine.

Germain, C. (1994). See my abuse: The shelter transition of battered women. In P. Munhall (Ed.), *In women's experience* (Vol. 1), pp. 201-231. New York: National League for Nursing Press.

Gilligan, C. (1993). *In a different voice: Psychological theory and women's development.* Cambridge, MA: Harvard University Press.

Glaser, B., & Strauss, A. (1967). *The discovery of grounded theory: Strategies for qualitative research.* New York: Aldine de Gruyter.

Gloerson, B., Kendall, J., Gray, P., McConnell, S., Turner, J., & Lewkowicz, J. (1993). The phenomena of doing well in people with AIDS. *Western Journal of Nursing Research, 15,* 44-58.

Goffman, E. (1993). *Stigma.* Englewood Cliffs, NJ: Prentice Hall.

Gregg, C., Robertus, J., & Stone, J. (1989). *The psychological aspects of chronic illness.* Springfield, IL: Thomas.

Gulley, L. (1991). *The etiology of anorexia: The client's viewpoint.* Unpublished dissertation, Vanderbilt University, Nashville, TN.

Haberman, B. (1996). Day-to-day demands of Parkinson's disease. *Western Journal of Nursing Research, 18,* 397-413.

Hainsworth, M. (1986). *An ethnographic study of women with multiple sclerosis using a symbolic interactionist approach.* Unpublished dissertation, University of Connecticut, Storrs, CT.

Hainsworth, M. (1994). Living with multiple sclerosis: The experience of chronic sorrow. *Journal of Neuroscience Nursing, 26,* 237-240.

Hall, J. (1994). How lesbians recognize and respond to alcohol problems: A theoretical model of problematization. *Advances in Nursing Science, 16,* (3), 46-63.

Hall, J., Roter, D., & Katz, N. (1988). Meta-analysis of correlates of provider behavior in medical encounters. *Medical Care, 26,* 657-675.

Hamilton, D. (1988). *Continual monitoring: A theoretical model of the weight loss maintenance process.* Unpublished dissertation, University of California at Berkeley.

Hawthorne, M. (1993). Women recovering from coronary artery bypass surgery. *Scholarly Inquiry for Nursing Practice, 7,* 223-248.

Henderson, D., Boyd, C., & Mieczkowski, T. (1994). Gender, relationships, and crack cocaine: A content analysis. *Research in Nursing & Health, 17,* 265-272.

Herman, J. (1992). *Trauma and recovery.* New York: BasicBooks.

Hesse-Biber, S. (1996). *Am I thin enough yet? The cult of thinness and the commercialization of identity.* New York: Oxford University Press.

Hinds, P., & Martin, J. (1988). Hopefulness and the self-sustaining process in adolescents with cancer. *Nursing Research, 37,* 336-340.

Howell, S. (1994). Natural/alternative health care practices used by women with chronic pain: Findings from a grounded theory research study. *Nurse Practitioner Forum, 5,* 98-105.

Hulbert, J. (1985). *Women addicted to alcohol and drugs: The recovery process.* Unpublished dissertation, University of Toronto, Toronto, Ontario, Canada.

Hutchinson, S. (1986). Chemically dependent nurses: The trajectory toward self-annihilation. *Nursing Research, 35,* 196-201.

Hutchinson, S. (1987). Toward self-integration: The recovery process of chemically dependent nurses. *Nursing Research, 36,* 339-343.

Jayne, R. (1993). *Self-regulation: Negotiating treatment regimens in insulin-dependent diabetes.* Unpublished dissertation, University of California at San Francisco.

Johnson, J., & Morse, J. (1990). Regaining control: The process of adjustment after myocardial infarction. *Heart & Lung, 19,* 126-135.

Johnson, R. (1990). Restructuring: An emerging theory on the process of losing weight. *Journal of Advanced Nursing, 15,* 1289-1296.

Johnston, K. (1996, August). *Physician gender and physician-patient relationships: A critical review of the literature* (Paper presented to American Sociological Association). San Francisco: University of California Department of Social and Behavioral Sciences.

Kagan, S. (1994). *Integrating cancer into a life mostly lived.* Unpublished dissertation, University of California at San Francisco.

Kasperkowski, U. (1991). *The body speaks: Seeking voice in a culture that silences.* Unpublished dissertation, University of Toronto, Toronto, Ontario, Canada.

Kearney, M. (1996). Reclaiming normal life: Mothers' stages of recovery from drug use. *Journal of Obstetric, Gynecologic, and Neonatal Nursing, 25,* 761-768.

Kearney, M., Murphy, S., & Rosenbaum, M. (1994). Mothering on crack cocaine: A grounded theory analysis. *Social Science and Medicine, 38,* 351-361.

Kelly-Powell, M. (1994). *Personalizing choices: The experiences of adults with potentially life-threatening conditions in their decision-making regarding treatment options.* Unpublished dissertation, University of Wisconsin, Milwaukee.

Kesselring, A. (1990). *The experienced body, when taken-for-grantedness falters: A phenomenological study of living with cancer.* Unpublished dissertation, University of California at San Francisco.

King, K., & Jensen, L. (1994). Preserving the self: Women having cardiac surgery. *Heart & Lung, 23,* 99-105.

Kleinman, A. (1988). *The illness narratives: Suffering, healing, and the human condition.* New York: Basic Books.

Klonoff, E., & Landrine, H. (1997). *Preventing misdiagnosis of women: A guide to physical disorders that have psychiatric symptoms.* Thousand Oaks, CA: Sage.

LaFramboise, B. (1993). *Finding voice: The psychosocial process of healing wounded women religious.* Unpublished dissertation, University of Alberta, Edmonton, Alberta, Canada.

Landenburger, K. (1989). A process of entrapment in and recovery from an abusive relationship. *Issues in Mental Health Nursing, 10,* 209-227.

Langner, S. (1995). The experience of being a woman with HIV/AIDS. In P. Munhall (Ed.), *In women's experience* (vol. 2), pp. 141-184. New York: National League for Nursing Press.

LaRosa, J., & Pinn, V. (1993). Gender bias in biomedical research. *Journal of the American Medical Women's Association, 48,* 145-151.

Lasker, R. (1997). *Medicine and public health: The power of collaboration.* New York: New York Academy of Medicine.

Lavizzo-Mourey, R., & Grisso, J. (1994). Health, health care, and women of color. In E. Friedman (Ed.), *An unfinished revolution: Women and health care in America,* pp. 47-63. New York: United Hospital Fund of New York.

Lee, T. (1991). *The Human Genome Project: Cracking the genetic code of life.* New York: Plenum.

Lemke, D., Pattison, J., Marshall, L., & Cowley, D. (1995). *Primary care of women.* Norwalk, CT: Appleton-Lange.

LeMone, P. (1993). Human sexuality in adults with insulin-dependent diabetes. *Image: Journal of Nursing Scholarship, 25,* 101-105.

Lempert, L. (1994). A narrative analysis of abuse. *Journal of Contemporary Ethnography, 22,* 411-441.

Leonard, K. (1990). *Women's experience of surviving invasive cervical cancer: Maintaining the self.* Unpublished dissertation, University of Alberta, Edmonton, Alberta, Canada.

Lewis, F., & Deal, L. (1995). Balancing our lives: A study of the married couple's experience with breast cancer recurrence. *Oncology Nursing Forum, 22,* 943-953.

Limandri, B. (1989). Disclosure of stigmatizing conditions: The discloser's perspective. *Archives of Psychiatric Nursing, 3,* 69-78.

Lombardi, J. (1982). *Growing up with violence: An analysis of retrospective accounts of female offspring.* Unpublished dissertation, University of Maryland, College Park, MD.

Lowery, C. (1994). *Life histories: Addiction and recovery of six Native American women.* Unpublished dissertation, University of Washington, Seattle.

Lubkin, I. (1995). *Chronic illness: Impact and intervention* (3rd ed.). Boston: Jones & Bartlett.

Maroni, J. (1986). *Alcoholic women: A study of their recovery process.* Unpublished dissertation, Catholic University of America, Washington, DC.

Marshak, L., & Seligman, M. (1993. *Counseling persons with physical disabilities: Theoretical and clinical perspectives.* Austin, TX: Pro-Ed.

Mastroianni, A., Faden, R., & Federman, D. (Eds.). (1994). *Women and health research: Vol. 1. Ethical and legal issues of including women in health studies.* Washington, DC: National Academy Press, Institute of Medicine.

Mathews, H., Lannin, D., & Mitchell, J. (1994). Coming to terms with advanced breast cancer: Black women's narratives from eastern North Carolina. *Social Science and Medicine, 38,* 789-800.

Mays, M., & Croake, J. (1997). *Treatment of depression in managed care.* New York: Brunner/Mazel.

McBarnette, L. (1996). African-American women. In M. Bayne-Smith (Ed.), *Race, gender, and health,* pp. 43-67. Thousand Oaks, CA: Sage.

Merritt-Gray, M., & Wuest, J. (1995). Counteracting abuse and breaking free: The process of leaving revealed through women's voices. *Health Care for Women International, 16,* 399-412.

Meyerowitz, B., & Hart, S. (1995). Women and cancer: Have assumptions about women limited our research agenda? In A. Stanton & S. Gallant (Eds.), *The psychology of women's health,* pp. 51-84. Washington, DC: American Psychological Association.

Montgomery, C. (1994). Swimming upstream: The strengths of women who survive homelessness. *Advances in Nursing Science, 16,* (3), 34-45.

Morrow, S. (1992). *Voices: Constructions of survival and coping by women survivors of child sexual abuse.* Unpublished dissertation, Arizona State University at Tempe.

Morrow, S., & Smith, M. (1995). Constructions of survival and coping by women who have survived childhood sexual abuse. *Journal of Counseling Psychology, 42,* 24-33.

Morse, J., & Carter, B. (1995). Strategies of enduring and the suffering of loss: Modes of comfort used by a resilient survivor. *Holistic Nursing Practice, 9,* (3), 38-52.

Morse, J., & Carter, B. (1996). The essence of enduring and expressions of suffering: The reformulation of self. *Scholarly Inquiry for Nursing Practice, 10,* 43-60.

Munhall, P. (1994). *In women's experience* (Vol. 1). New York: National League for Nursing Press.

Munhall, P. (1995). *In women's experience* (Vol. 2). New York: National League for Nursing Press.

Munhall, P., & Boyd, C. (1993). *Nursing research: A qualitative perspective* (2nd ed.). New York: National League for Nursing Press.

Nelson, A. (1990). Patients' perceptions of a spinal cord injury unit. *SCI Nursing, 7,* 44-63.

Newman, K. (1993). Giving up: Shelter experiences of battered women. *Public Health Nursing, 10,* 108-113.

Parratt, J. (1994). The experience of childbirth for survivors of incest. *Midwifery, 10,* 26-39.

Payne, S. (1990). Coping with palliative chemotherapy. *Journal of Advanced Nursing, 15,* 652-658.

Persic, A. (1993). *An exploration of bulimia and coping.* Unpublished masters thesis, University of Calgary, Calgary, Alberta, Canada.

Pilowsky, J. (1993). *The price of a wife is thirteen cents: An exploration of abused Spanish-speaking women.* Unpublished dissertation, University of Toronto, Toronto, Ontario, Canada.

Price, M. (1993). An experiential model of learning diabetes self-management. *Qualitative Health Research, 3,* 29-54.

Quinn, A., Barton, J., & Magilvy, J. (1995). Weathering the storm: Metaphors and stories of living with multiple sclerosis. *Rehabilitation Nursing Research, 4,* 19-27.

Rankin, S. (1992). Psychosocial adjustments of coronary artery disease patients and their spouses: Nursing implications. *Nursing Clinics of North America, 27,* 271-284.

Reast, R. (1993). *Experiences of women who have had myocardial infarction treated with angioplasty.* Unpublished masters thesis, Texas Tech, Health Sciences Center, Lubbock, TX.

Register, C. (1987). *Living with chronic illness: Days of patience and passion.* New York: Free Press.

Rosser, S. (1994). *Women's health: Missing from U.S. medicine.* Bloomington: Indiana University Press.

Schaefer, K. (1995). Struggling to maintain balance: A study of women living with fibromyalgia. *Journal of Advanced Nursing, 21,* 95-102.

Seals, B., Sowell, R., Demi, A., Moneyham, L., Cohen, L., & Guillory, J. (1995). Falling through the cracks: Social service concerns of women infected with HIV. *Qualitative Health Research, 5,* 496-515.

Soderberg, S., Lundman, B., & Norberg, A. (1997). Living with fibromyalgia: Sense of coherence, perception of well-being, and stress in daily life. *Research in Nursing & Health, 20,* 495-503.

Stanton, A. (1995). Psychology of women's health: Barriers and pathways to knowledge. In A. Stanton & S. Gallant (Eds.), *The psychology of women's health,* pp. 3-21. Washington, DC: American Psychological Association.

Stevens, P. (1996). Struggles with symptoms: Women's narratives of managing HIV illness. *Journal of Holistic Nursing, 14,* 142-161.

Strauss, A. (1975). *Chronic illness and the quality of life.* St. Louis, MO: C.V. Mosby.

Strauss, A. (1987). *Qualitative analysis for social scientists.* Cambridge, UK: Cambridge University Press.

Strauss, A., & Corbin, J. (1988). *Shaping a new health care system: The explosion of chronic illness as a catalyst for change.* San Francisco: Jossey-Bass.

Strauss, A., & Corbin, J. (1990). *Basics of qualitative research: Grounded theory procedures and techniques.* Newbury Park, CA: Sage.

Stuart, E., & Campbell, J. (1989). Assessment of patterns of dangerousness with battered women. *Issues in Mental Health Nursing, 10,* 245-260.

Stuifbergen, A., & Rogers, S. (1997). The experience of fatigue and strategies of self-care among persons with multiple sclerosis. *Applied Nursing Research, 10,* 2-10.

Swanson, J., & Chenitz, C. (1993). Regaining a valued self: The process of adaptation to living with genital herpes. *Qualitative Health Research, 3,* 270-297.

Taggart, L., McCammon, S., Allred, L., Horner, R., & May, H. (1993). Effect of patient and physician gender on prescriptions for psychotropic drugs. *Journal of Women's Health, 2,* 353-357.

Taylor, S., & Aspinwall, L. (1990). Psychological aspects of chronic illness. In P. Costa & G. VandenBos (Eds.), *Psychological aspects of serious illness: Chronic conditions, fatal diseases, and clinical care,* pp. 7-60. Washington, DC: American Psychological Association.

Telch, C., & Telch, M. (1986). Group coping skills interaction and supportive group therapy for cancer patients: A comparison of strategies. *Journal of Consulting and Clinical Psychology, 54,* 802-808.

Ternulf Nyhlin, K. (1991). The fine balancing act of managing diabetes. *Scandinavian Journal of Caring Sciences, 5,* 187-194.

Thorne, S. (1990). Constructive noncompliance in chronic illness. *Holistic Nursing Practice, 5,* 62-69.

Thorne, S. (1993). *Negotiating health care: The social context of chronic illness.* Newbury Park, CA: Sage.

Ulrich, Y. (1993). What helped most in leaving spouse abuse: Implications for interventions. *AWHONN's Clinical Issues, 4,* 385-390.

Vourakis, C. (1989). *The process of recovery for women in Alcoholics Anonymous: Seeking groups "like me."* Unpublished dissertation, University of California at San Francisco.

Weisman, C., & Cassard, S. (1994). Health consequences of exclusion or underrepresentation of women in clinical studies (I). In A. Mastroianni, R. Faden, & D. Federman (Eds.), *Women and health research: Vol. 2. Workshop and commissioned papers,* pp. 35-40. Washington, DC: National Academy Press, Institute of Medicine.

Welch, H. (1996). Nurse midwives as primary care providers for women. *Clinical Nurse Specialist, 10,* 121-124, 143.

West, C. (1984). *Routine complications: Troubles with talk between doctors and patients*. Bloomington: Indiana University Press.

Westra, B. (1991). *Getting back to living life: Older adults' experience at home after hospitalization*. Unpublished dissertation, University of Wisconsin at Milwaukee.

Westra, B. (1993, January). Elders' experiences at home after hospital discharge. *Minnesota Nurses' Association Accent, 1*, 9.

Wiener, C., & Dodd, M. (1993). Coping amid uncertainty: An illness trajectory perspective. *Scholarly Inquiry for Nursing Practice, 7*, 17-31.

Wilson, H., Hutchinson, S., & Holzemer, W. (1997). Salvaging quality of life in ethnically diverse patients with advanced HIV/AIDS. *Qualitative Health Research, 7*, 75-97.

Woodhouse, L. (1992). Women with jagged edges: Voices from a culture of substance abuse. *Qualitative Health Research, 2*, 262-281.

Young-Mason, J. (1997). *The patient's voice: Experiences of illness*. Philadelphia: F. A. Davis.

Index

About the Author

Margaret H. Kearney, RN (Ph.D., University of California at San Francisco), is a certified women's health nurse practitioner and an associate professor of nursing at Boston College, in Chestnut Hill, MA. She is interested in the self-care experiences of pregnant and parenting women and has conducted a number of qualitative studies with addicted and recovering women using the grounded theory approach. Her current research focuses on the impact of violence during pregnancy, on nursing support of socially high-risk pregnant women and mothers, and on qualitative approaches to meta-analysis.